Anna
Del Conte
Vegetables
all'Italiana

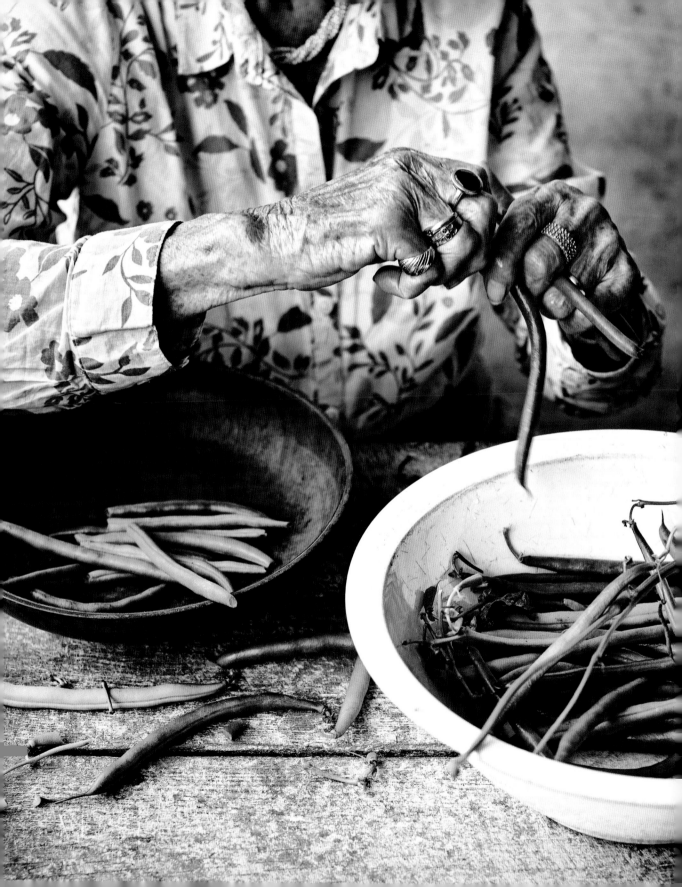

Anna Del Conte
Vegetables all'Italiana

PAVILION

First published in the United Kingdom in 2018 by
Pavilion
43 Great Ormond Street
London
WC1N 3HZ

ISBN 978-1-91159-544-1

A CIP catalogue record for this book is available from the British Library.

10 9 8 7 6 5 4 3 2 1

Reproduction by Mission, Hong Kong
Printed and bound by 1010 Printing International Ltd, China

This book can be ordered direct from the publisher at
www.pavilionbooks.com

This page: Zucchine al Forno al Sapor di Mentuccia (see page 184)

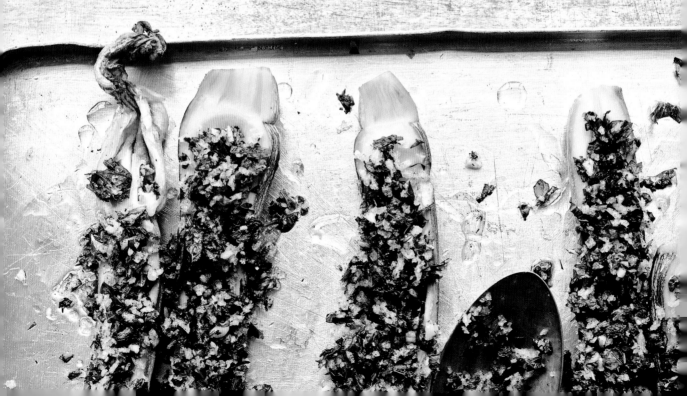

Verdure Vegetables 7

Aglio Garlic 10

Asparago Asparagus 13

Barbabietola Beetroot 17

Broccoli e Broccoletti Broccoli and Broccoletti 22

Carciofo Globe Artichoke 26

Cardo Cardoon 30

Carota Carrot 32

Cavolfiore Cauliflower 38

Cavolini di Bruxelles Brussels Sprouts 46

Cavolo Cabbage 49

Ceci Chickpeas 59

Cetriolo Cucumber 62

Cipolla Onion 63

Coste Swiss Chard 69

Fagiolini Green Beans 71

Fagioli Beans 77

Fave Broad Beans 77

Finocchio Fennel 86

Funghi Mushrooms 92

Lattuga Lettuce 95

Lenticchie Lentils 98

Melanzana Aubergine 103

Patata Potato 112

Peperone Pepper 122

Piselli Peas 130

Pomodoro Tomato 136

Porro Leek 141

Puntarelle Puntarelle 146

Radicchio Radicchio 148

Rapa Turnip 152

Rapanello Radish 154

Scorzonera Black Salsify 156

Sedano Celery 157

Sedano di Verona Celeriac 160

Spinaci Spinach 163

Taccola Mangetout 175

Topinambour Jerusalem Artichoke 177

Zucca Pumpkin and Squash 178

Zucchina Courgette 182

Sauces and Mixed Vegetable Dishes 192

Index 204

Acknowledgements 208

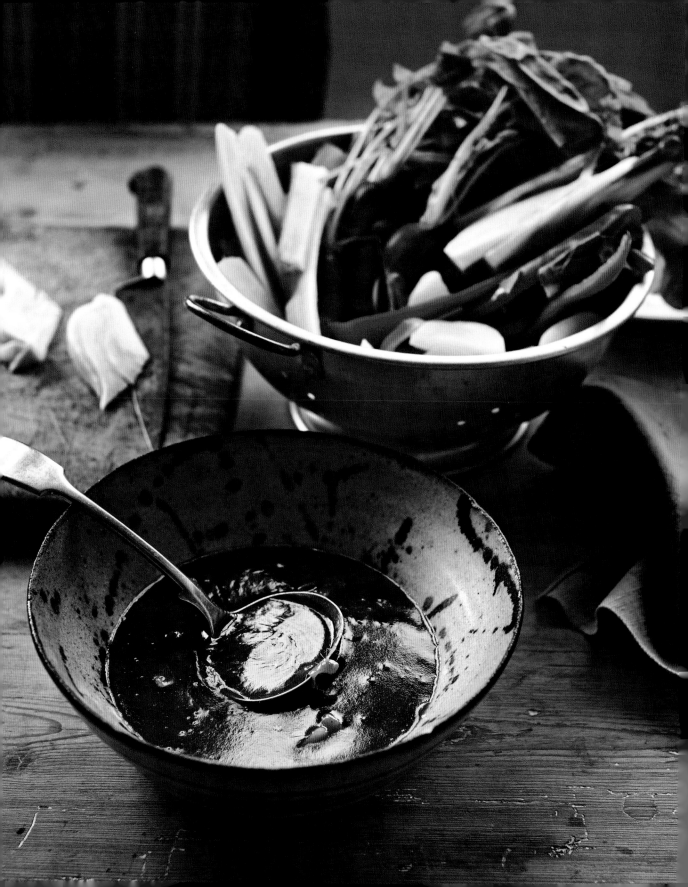

Verdure
Vegetables

This is a book on *verdure* or vegetables, where vegetables are treated with all the due reverence that they are in Italy, where they are never thought of just as an accompaniment to the main meat or the fish dish, even when they are served alongside.

As soon as I set foot in this country over half a century ago, I realised that the English view was that vegetables were just something healthy one should eat with the meat or the fish course. I know that at that time most people were not at all interested in food of any kind, and vegetables were certainly at the bottom of the list. I was lucky enough to land, as an au-pair, with a family where good food was appreciated and enjoyed. Kitty, my hostess, was a good cook and she excelled at baking – at making pies and puddings, cakes and biscuits – all extremely English. But when it came to vegetables, Kitty usually just boiled them, 'though not "overso" ' and that was it. They were very good vegetables, most of them coming to the kitchen straight from the large vegetable garden that her one-legged gardener was lovingly looking after. Occasionally, Kitty would make a white sauce to go with the vegetables. Otherwise they came to the table totally 'naked'.

One day Kitty asked me if I could cook the carrots that were on the kitchen table, just dug from the ground. 'Yes, of course,' and out I reached for the frying pan, a small onion, the bottle of the precious olive oil and the pack of margarine – the rationed butter was kept for spreading on toast and bread. I scrubbed and washed the carrots and cut them in thin discs; and chopped a little of the onion. I put one or two tablespoons of oil and a lump of margarine in the pan and heated it. Then I added the onion and, when it was just turning a golden colour I chucked in the carrots and cooked them gently while adding a little stock every now and then. The stock was most probably chicken, from one of the local hens – Kitty's, the gardener's, or some neighbours', since everybody had hens at that time. Those carrots were one of my greatest culinary triumphs and yet they were simply cooked, *all'italiana*, in the everyday Italian way.

The vegetable scenario is now totally different. Vegetables of all sorts are widely available the whole year round, even too much so. I prefer to eat vegetables when they are in season as I was brought up to do. Now, for instance, I am writing this book in March, which is probably the least vegetable season-friendly month of the year. And in my larder – living in an old house in the country, I still have the luxury of a larder – there are a leek, half a Savoy cabbage, as well as the usual potatoes, carrots and celery. However, no courgettes, peppers or aubergines. I might have a tomato or two but certainly not for eating in salad, more for cooking whenever I need it. The other stand-by in my kitchen is frozen petits pois, which so often has saved me from a meal without vegetables. And, I nearly forgot, a fennel bulb. I don't know why I can eat fennel out of season; probably because they are never 'in season' in this country, since they can't be cultivated here because of the weather.

The 132 recipes in this book will show just how much you can do with a vegetable. Some of these recipes are quick and easy, some are more demanding and complicated, but all are worth having a go. There are no pasta sauces and no risotto recipes here, because in these instances the main ingredient would be the pasta or the rice, not the vegetable.

It would be fair to say that most of the recipes are suitable for vegetarians and even the non-vegetarian recipes can easily become vegetarian with a slight tweak of the ingredients. For instance, in the recipe for *Broccoli in Padella con la Pancetta* or Sautéed Broccoli with Pancetta (see page 23), you can omit the pancetta and add instead a little more oil; and there are a few recipes containing anchovies or tuna, or perhaps a little meat stock, which can be adapted if necessary, but, for the most part, the recipes are vegetarian.

Most of the recipes are for four people. However, some recipes are for more because the dish can only be made successfully in larger quantities. The serving quantities

Left: Bagna Caôda (see page 30)

can only be a guidance because other factors have a role to play. Are the people who are going to eat that dish young or old? Is that their only meal of the day? What is coming before or after the dish in question? I usually err on the side of plenty; I prefer to have left-overs, than to see my guests scraping the last spoonful of the dish.

When you follow a recipe, use just one system of measures – metric, imperial or cups – all through the recipe. All spoons are meant to be level. 1 tablespoon = 15 ml, 1 teaspoon = 5 ml. A set of measuring spoons is a great help to a cook. A set includes 5 spoons which measure from 'a pinch' to 1 tablespoon.

My recipes are only a guide. Read them, cook them once or twice and then give them a slight twist, your own signature. Make them part of you, as your food is. You will enjoy cooking far more if you don't stick literally to the gospel of a recipe book. However, it is important to pay attention to the proportions of the ingredients used. This will teach you to achieve the 'Italian flavour', and having learnt that, you will no longer need to follow a recipe slavishly. I would also stress that good cooking requires precision, care and patience. Creativity comes later, just as in any other art.

Notes for the reader

My English friends have suggested that I should include some of the little points that crop up in my conversations with them and which, they say, are often unfamiliar to the non-professional cook. So let's start by giving an explanation of some of the Italian culinary terms I use.

Battuto is a pounded mixture (the word comes from *battere* – to beat or pound). The *battuto* is the basis of most dishes, from a pasta sauce to a bean soup. Nowadays a mixture of olive oil and butter are used instead of pork fat, with possibly a little pancetta or prosciutto. When I add pancetta or prosciutto I use a food processor, which does an excellent job in a whizz. A *battuto* usually becomes a *soffritto*, except when it is added *a crudo* (in the raw state) to a sauce or a soup.

Soffritto is the *battuto* which has been fried, or actually 'under-fried', which is what the word means. The *battuto* is sautéed in a saucepan or a frying pan over a gentle heat until the onion is soft. When using garlic, this should be added to the onion later, when the onion is nearly done, or the garlic will become too dark by the time the onion is soft. Only when the *battuto* contains pancetta or fatty prosciutto can the garlic be added at the same time. A well-made *soffritto* is fundamental to the final taste of the dish.

Here are some of my tips, arranged in alphabetical order.

BUTTER
I always use unsalted butter – it has a more delicate flavour and can be heated to a higher temperature than salted butter. To heat butter to a higher temperature without burning, I add some olive oil.

CHILLI
In most regions of Italy chillies are a new ingredient and still used parsimoniously. The kind used are the small, dried ones, reputedly among the hottest of them all. I suggest that you experiment with what you buy, keeping in mind that Italian dishes are never very hot, the chilli being considered a flavouring to blend with others and not provide an overriding fire.

DRIED PORCINI
Depending on the porcini, these should be soaked for about 1 hour before use. If they are beautiful, large, fresh-looking slices they will only need 20 minutes or so, but if they are small, dried-up pieces they will need a longer soaking time.

EGGS
Some recipes require specific egg sizes. Where no size is specified you can use either medium or large.

FORK OR SPOON
Use a fork to stir sautéeing potatoes, carrots, courgettes and other vegetables. Spoons tend to break them.

LEMONS
I prefer to use unwaxed fruits. The wax sprayed on the fruit is toxic, and it does not wash off easily. If you cannot find unwaxed fruits, put your lemons in a sink of very hot water and scrub hard.

OLIVE OIL

When you use olive oil as a base for a *soffritto* together with butter, you do not need to use extra virgin olive oil. Any plain olive oil will do, as it has less flavour and is lighter. I use plain olive oil or groundnut oil for deep frying, as it can be heated to the high temperature needed.

PANCETTA

Pancetta, from the belly of a pig, is a similar cut to streaky bacon, but is differently cured. You can buy pancetta, smoked or unsmoked, already diced, in vacuum packs. This is ideal for a *battuto*.

PROSCIUTTO

If you can, ask for the knuckle of a prosciutto, which is usually half the price of the prosciutto itself. This end piece has the right proportion of lean meat to fat, necessary for *battuti*, sauce bases or for stuffing or larding. Ask the butcher to cut off all the rind (you can keep this for flavouring a pulse soup or a stew), and then cut the meat into chunks and keep them in the freezer. For cooking I prefer to use prosciutto di San Daniele rather than prosciutto di Parma because it has a stronger flavour.

SALT AND PEPPER

Salt enhances the flavour of food. Use good sea salt, such as Maldon, which is best for cooking and for your health. The right amount of salt – a personal choice – should be added at the beginning or during the cooking, in time for it to dissolve properly and flavour all the dish. If added at the table, not only is the result unsatisfactory, but also more salt usually has to be added to achieve the right seasoning. Always add salt to the water before you add pasta, rice or vegetables.

Pepper is used more sparingly in Italian cooking than in many other cuisines. Use freshly ground black pepper if possible.

STOCK

Add the outside leaf of an onion to impart a lovely golden colour to your chicken stock. Italian cooks use fresh stock or bouillon cubes in quite a few dishes. This is not an aberration. Stock cubes in Italy are less strong than those sold in other countries. Many stock cubes are now available that contain a minimum of monosodium glutamate or none at all, and they are really quite good. Remember that stock cubes are salty, so add less salt. I also use Marigold Swiss vegetable bouillon powder.

TOMATOES

Keep fresh tomatoes out of the refrigerator, preferably on a sunny windowsill. They will become tastier and their all-too-often leathery skins will soften. For cooking I prefer to use good-quality canned tomatoes which have more flavour.

VEGETABLES

This is one of my hobby horses. When I came to England in the 1950s, the vegetables were cooked – boiled – to a mush. Then came nouvelle cuisine, and now the vegetables served in many restaurants are simply raw. For us Italians, crunchy French beans or al dente asparagus are anathema, and even worse are crunchy turnips, lentils or artichokes.

It is not possible to give a precise cooking time for vegetables, since it depends on their quality and freshness. It also depends on whether the vegetable has been grown in proper earth or in a hydroponic culture, in which case it will cook very quickly indeed. Also remember that the cooking time for stewing vegetables, in very little liquid, is longer than for boiling in plenty of water or for frying. Carrots, for instance, will be cooked in 10 minutes maximum in boiling water, but will take longer, even cut into sticks, if you cook them in oil and/or butter with a little stock or water added gradually.

VINEGAR

I am always surprised that so much has been written on the finer points of olive oils, yet so little about the importance of good wine vinegar. A salad dressed even with the best extra virgin olive oil can be ruined by a second-rate vinegar. You will know a vinegar is good by its price – good vinegar is not cheap, because it comes from a decent wine. The process of making the vinegar must not be accelerated by the addition of chemicals. Wine vinegar is the only one traditionally used in Italy. Red and white wine vinegar differ mainly in colour, the flavour being similar.

Aglio
Garlic

Garlic has been used in Italy since Roman times, but always with moderation and discrimination. During the Renaissance it was considered food for the peasant and rarely appeared on the grand tables of princes. In fact, it hardly appeared in Italian cookery books of the 19th and first half of the 20th century. Pellegrino Artusi, the great 19th-century cookery writer who wrote the most popular cookery book in Italy for decades, *La Scienza in Cucina e l'Arte di Mangiar Bene* (Science in the Kitchen and the Art of Eating Well) (1891), does not use a lot of garlic, nor does Ada Boni, the author of *Il Talismano della Felicità* (1929), two of the very few cookery books I consult regularly. The very moderate use of garlic in Italy was partly due to the pungent smell that can linger on for hours on the breath of the person who has eaten it. I well remember the buses in Rome – you squeeze in and are assailed by the smell of garlic mixed with human sweat. Not a Dior creation. I still remember my mother saying, 'You can't have this salad; it has too much garlic and tomorrow you are going to have lunch with So and So'. Now people do not seem to mind at all the smell of garlic and even the finicky northern Milanese eat it with relish.

Garlic has very powerful beneficial properties: it protects against the cold and flu virus, it helps reduce blood pressure and postpones the onset of Alzheimers and dementia, and might even have a beneficial effect against bowel cancer. Virgil wrote that garlic has the right properties to maintain the strength of the harvest reapers. And in the Middle Ages it was believed that it could protect virgin girls from vampire bites. You only had to tie a string of garlic to the bed frame and you were safe.

There are two main varieties of this perennial plant: white garlic and pink garlic; the pink variety, which is less common, is slightly sweeter. Fresh garlic, in season in late spring and summer, is slightly less pungent than dried garlic. To reduce the pungency of older, dried garlic, you can remove the germ (the tiny pale green shoot inside the clove). Another method, used mostly in northern Italy where the pungency of garlic is less appreciated, is to steep the cloves in hot milk for 30 minutes or more before using. This is often done in Piedmont to prepare the garlic cloves used in their famous sauce – *Bagna Caôda* (see page 30).

Garlic is used more in southern Italy than in the north; the cuisine of the south is based more on oil and tomato, which combine better with the flavour of garlic. Usually garlic is used as an additional flavouring and not as a main ingredient. In only one sauce, *Agliata* (see page 12) is garlic the prime ingredient. It is also a main ingredient in the classic dish *spaghetti olio, aglio e peperoncino* (spaghetti with oil, garlic and chilli).

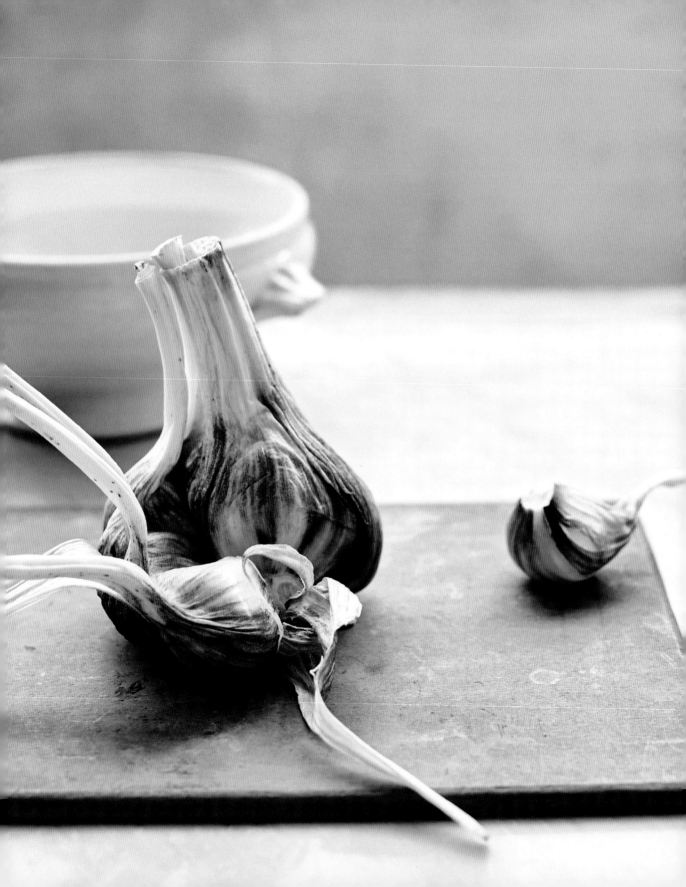

Agliata
Garlic Sauce

This is one of Liguria's classic sauces – others are basil pesto and walnut sauce. It is the sauce traditionally served with boiled meat of any sort and poached or boiled fish. As with mayonnaise, the oil must be added very slowly or the sauce will split. Some cooks add Dijon mustard at the end, as in this recipe; I like to use English mustard powder – it is stronger and I find the taste combines better with the other ingredients. If using, add 1 tsp of English mustard powder instead of Dijon mustard.

Serves 6–8

50g/1¾oz crustless sourdough white bread

5 tbsp white wine vinegar

4 fat garlic cloves, coarsely chopped

100–125ml/3½–4fl oz/scant ½–¾ cup vegetable stock or water and vegetable bouillon powder

100ml/3½fl oz/scant ½ cup extra virgin olive oil

1 tbsp Dijon mustard

Sea salt

Break the bread up into small pieces and put in a saucepan. Add the vinegar, garlic, salt and about three-quarters of the stock or water and put the pan on a low heat. Bring to a simmer and cook very, very gently. To be safe, I use a flame diffuser. Let the sauce bubble gently away for 10 minutes, but keep an eye on it and add a little more stock if it begins to catch. If you finish the stock before the 10 minutes is up, add a little hot water.

Transfer the sauce into the small bowl of a food processor, turn the machine on and begin to add the oil, drop by drop. As with making mayonnaise, you have to be extra careful in the early stages of adding the oil. After you have added the first half, you can add the oil a little more quickly.

Transfer the sauce to a bowl, mix in the mustard and then taste and adjust the salt, if necessary.

Asparago
Asparagus

Beloved by both the Romans and Renaissance princes, asparagus is still considered a luxury food. Bartolomeo Scappi was chef to two popes in the second half of the 16th century and was for cooking what Michelangelo was for the arts. In his great book *Opera dell'Arte del Ben Cucinare* Scappi rates the properties of this vegetable very highly and, among others, gives a recipe for it to be cooked in meat stock and then served in the stock with bits of the meat. In the late 19th century Artusi also cooks asparagus in meat stock and then serves it dressed with butter and 'a gentle flowering of Parmesan', my translation.

In Italy asparagus is still simply served dressed with melted butter and grated Parmesan, as well as with olive oil and lemon juice.

The most popular varieties of Italian asparagus are the big, white Bianchi di Bassano from Veneto, the green of Piedmont or Romagna and the purple of Naples. Personally I prefer green asparagus to the other varieties, as I like them simply dressed *alla milanese* (see page 14) or *all'agro*, with mild extra virgin olive oil and lemon juice.

Favourite asparagus dishes of northern Italy are *risotto agli asparagi* and *frittata agli asparagi*, both made with butter flavoured with chopped onion, not garlic.

To prepare asparagus, take a spear and bend it. It will snap just at the correct point that separates the woody stalk from the spear. Discard the woody stalks or save them to make a soup. Wash the spears and drain thoroughly. The asparagus is now ready to be cooked.

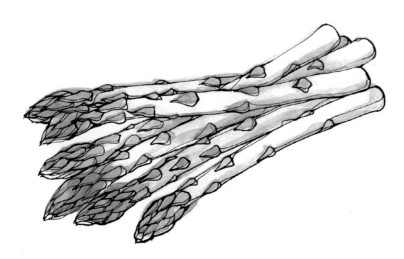

Asparagi alla Milanese
Asparagus with Eggs and Grated Parmesan

This dish takes me back to a spring meal of my childhood in Milan. I loved the dish mainly because it was one of the very few foods I was allowed to eat with my hands. I loved dragging the asparagus spears along the plate, gently breaking the egg yolk, and then turning the spear in the yolk and quickly catching it in my open mouth.

The asparagus we ate then were the green asparagus of Piedmont, which are supposed to be the best, not the fat, white variety from Bassano in Veneto, which my mother thought were not as good – and I agree with her.

In Milan leeks are also called 'the asparagus of the poor' because they are so much cheaper than asparagus. This recipe works perfectly using leeks (when it is called *porri alla milanese*). Use only the white part of the leeks – if large, cut the bulbs in half – and cook them in boiling, salted water for 5 minutes. Drain and dry very thoroughly. Place each portion on individual plates and then proceed as for the recipe below from the last paragraph.

Serves 4

750g/1lb 10oz green asparagus

Sea salt

60g/2¼oz/4 tbsp unsalted butter

6 tbsp freshly grated Parmesan

1 tbsp olive oil

8 eggs

Prepare the asparagus (see page 13) and tie the spears into four bundles in two places, one at the top just under the tips and one at the other end.

Bring a large sauté pan full of water to the boil, add 1 tbsp of salt and plunge in the asparagus bundles. Cook until the spears are just tender when pricked by the point of a knife, which will take from 3–6 minutes. It is difficult to specify the cooking time required as it depends on the freshness of the asparagus, how thick the spears are and how tender you like your asparagus. I like mine cooked until they just gently bend when you lift them up to bring to your mouth; but you might like yours more al dente. When the asparagus are cooked to your liking, drain and dry them thoroughly, place each bundle on a plate and keep them warm in a low oven while you cook the eggs.

Melt about three-quarters of the butter in a large non-stick frying pan and when the butter begins to turn golden, pour it over the asparagus. Sprinkle with the Parmesan. Put the plates back in the oven.

Melt the remaining butter and the olive oil in the same pan and then gently break in the eggs, one next to the other. Turn the heat down and cook the eggs until the white is just firm, but the yolk is still runny. Using a fish slice, slide 2 eggs onto each plate of asparagus and sprinkle with a little salt. Bring the plates to the table. In Milan no pepper is added, but you can obviously add some if you prefer.

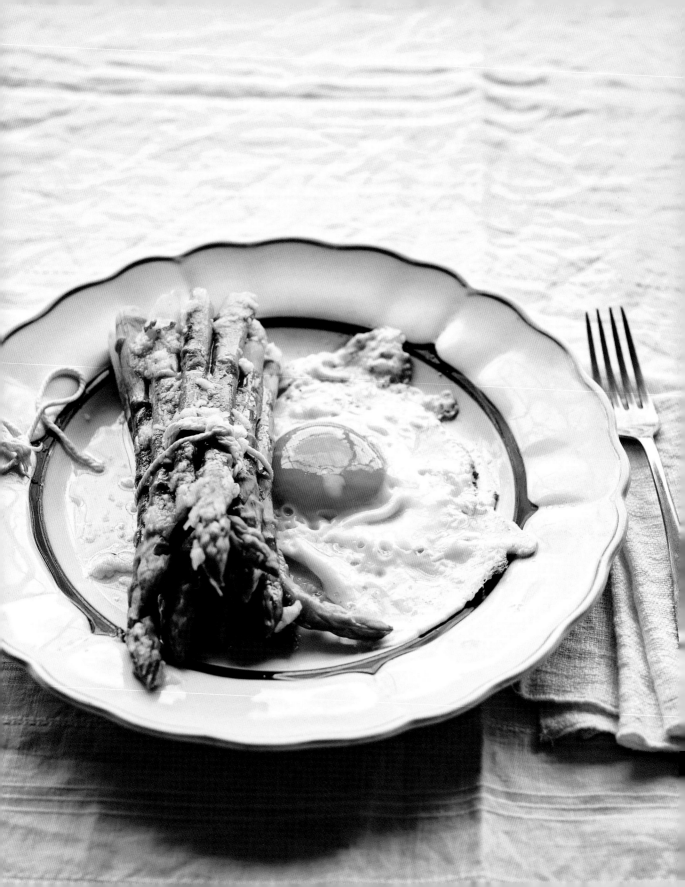

Fagottini di Asparagi col Prosciutto
Baked Asparagus Wrapped in Prosciutto

This is the only way I like baked asparagus. The prosciutto protects the spears and allows them to cook properly without becoming too brittle; besides, it gives the asparagus a deliciously gentle piggy flavour.

Try to buy asparagus spears all the same size and prosciutto with as much fat as possible.

Serves 4

750g/1lb 10oz asparagus
8 slices prosciutto, about 200g/7oz
25g/1oz/1½ tbsp unsalted butter
Freshly ground black pepper
Oil for the baking sheet

Heat the oven to 160°C Fan/180°C/350°F/Gas Mark 4.

Prepare the asparagus (see page 13). Divide the spears into 4 equal bundles according to their thickness.

Unwrap the prosciutto and place 2 slices on a chopping board. Place a bundle of asparagus on top of the prosciutto slices. Dot a little of the butter here and there among the spears and sprinkle with a little pepper, but not salt as the prosciutto should give the asparagus enough saltiness. Wrap the prosciutto neatly around the asparagus. Do the same with the other 3 bundles of asparagus.

Brush a baking sheet with a little oil, place the bundles on it and bake for 30 minutes. Test to see if the asparagus are done, by inserting the point of a small knife into the thickest part of a spear. It should go in easily. I find 30 minutes to be the minimum time they need. More often they take 40 minutes, but you might prefer asparagus more al dente than I do.

When the asparagus are done to your liking, transfer them to individual plates and serve them as they are, just by themselves. If you want to make the dish more filling, serve with some steamed, small new potatoes rolled in plenty of butter and sprinkled with a few chopped chives.

Barbabietola
Beetroot

This lovely red root is mostly grown and eaten in northern Italy. The Romans were fond of beetroots, but used the leaves rather than the roots. I do eat the leaves, too, and find them good. To use the leaves, remove the stalks, wash the leaves and boil them in a little water and 1 tsp of salt until tender. Drain well and squeeze out the liquid. Chop the leaves and dress them with a little olive oil and lemon juice, sometimes adding a few anchovy fillets, chopped if you prefer, a thinly sliced garlic clove and a pinch of chilli flakes. I sometimes also sauté them in butter, and use them as I would spinach leaves.

In Italy beetroots are usually sold already cooked, just simply boiled, as was done decades ago when I was a child. My mother used to buy them from the man who cooked them there in the street at the corner of Via Montenapoleone and Via Borgospesso in the cauldron which sat on his tricycle. As well as boiled beetroots, he also sold boiled onions, big juicy ones which I carried home wrapped in newspaper, holding them in my hands under my nose, enjoying two pleasures at the same time: the smell and the heat. I still love beetroots and here in Dorset I buy them raw and cook them at home. I usually boil them, because I find it easier to judge when they are cooked than if I bake them.

To boil beetroots, put them in a large saucepan, cover with cold water to come about 5cm/2in above their level. Add 1 tbsp of salt and bring the water to the boil. Turn the heat down to simmer and cook until the point of a small knife can enter easily into the middle of a beetroot. If your beetroots are of different size, test the smallest root after 20–25 minutes. Do not lift the beetroots out of the water until they are properly cooked. Remove the skins as soon as the beetroots are cool enough to handle and cut into slices or cubes, depending on the recipe.

Insalata di Barbabietole, Patate e Scalogno
Beetroot, Potato and Shallot Salad

Beetroots used to appear regularly on our table in Milan during the autumn and winter, as I am sure they still do nowadays. When I was young, vegetables had seasons, and beetroots were one of the few vegetables that could be served in a salad during the winter months. They were often served dressed with oil and vinegar just by themselves or with other cooked vegetables, as in this recipe.

Serves 6

3 medium waxy or salad potatoes

400g/14oz small round shallots

*4 medium beetroots (beet), cooked and
    peeled*

4 tbsp extra virgin olive oil

3 tbsp balsamic vinegar

1 tbsp Dijon mustard

*Sea salt and freshly ground black
    pepper*

*15–25g/½–1oz/1 cup mint leaves,
    coarsely chopped*

Wash the potatoes and put them in a pan. Cover with cold water, add 1 tbsp of salt and bring to the boil. Cook until done, but still just firm. Drain and peel as soon as they are cool enough to handle. Set aside to become cold – potatoes become firmer when cold and they don't break so easily. Cut into small cubes and add to a salad bowl.

While the potatoes are cooking, wash the shallots under cold water, put them in a pan with 1 tbsp of salt and cover with water. Bring to the boil and cook them for about 20 minutes, until just done, depending on size. Drain and then peel them when they are cool enough to handle. It will be quite easy – just squeeze the inside of the shallot and it will pop out leaving the layer of skin between your thumb and finger. Add to the salad bowl.

Cut the beetroots into cubes the same size as the potatoes and add to the salad bowl.

Pour the oil into a small bowl and beat in the vinegar, mustard and salt and pepper to taste. Spoon the sauce over the vegetables and mix gently. Sprinkle with the mint.

Sometimes, if I am in the mood of 'I like to paint what I eat', I take a large, round dish rather than a salad bowl, pile the potatoes in the middle surround them with the beetroot and spoon the dressing over the top.

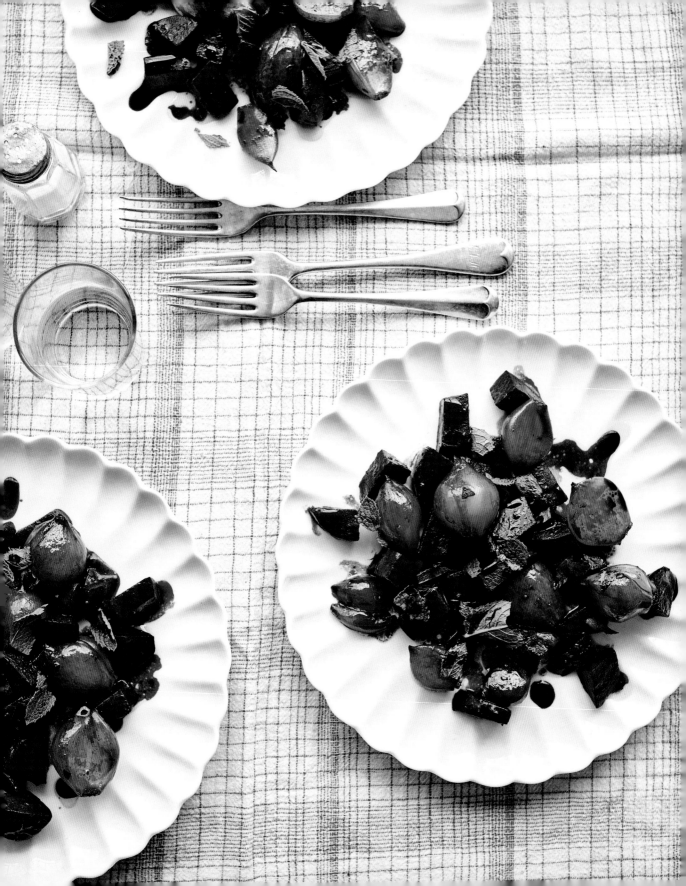

Barbabietole Saltate alle Erbe
Sautéed Beetroot with Herbs and Garlic

In early September my daughter's allotment seems to be able to produce nothing but beetroots. I even found time this year to make beetroot gnocchi, because I was becoming bored of the usual beetroot salad or beetroot mixed with yogurt. Then I remembered a beetroot dish my mother used to cook in Milan during the winter. At that time, the only herbs available in winter were parsley and sage. But now I make this recipe with a range of different herbs and the result is even more delicious.

Serves 4–6

500g/1lb 2oz beetroots (beet), cooked and peeled

20g/1¾oz/1½ tbsp unsalted butter

1 tbsp olive oil

2 garlic cloves, crushed

15–25g/½–1oz/1 cup mixed herbs, such as parsley, marjoram, sage, chives, chervil, chopped

Juice of ½ unwaxed lemon

Sea salt and freshly ground black pepper

Cut the beetroots into 1cm/½in slices. If the beetroots are large, cut them in half before you slice them.

Heat the butter in a frying pan, add the beetroots and gently fry for 5 minutes, turning them over frequently. Transfer the beetroots to a serving dish and keep warm.

In the same frying pan, heat the oil with the garlic and when the garlic is starting to colour add the herbs. Sauté over a gentle heat for 2 minutes and then remove the garlic and discard. Spoon the *salsina* over the beetroots. Season with the lemon juice and salt and pepper to taste and serve hot.

Gnocchi di Barbabietola
Beetroot Gnocchi

These gnocchi are as pretty in their pinky guise as they are delicious in their earthy flavour. Like potato gnocchi, and even more so, these pink gnocchi are best simply dressed with melted butter flavoured with sage leaves and garlic. Try to buy potatoes all of the same size.

Serves 6
450g/1lb waxy, slightly older potatoes

150g/5½oz beetroots (beet), cooked
   and peeled

500–600g/1lb 2oz–1lb 5 oz/
   4–4¾ cups flour

Plenty of freshly grated Parmesan

Sea salt and freshly ground black
   pepper

For the dressing
50g/1¾oz/4 tbsp unsalted butter

6 sage leaves, torn into small pieces

2 garlic cloves, crushed

Wash the potatoes and cook in plenty of boiling, salted water until tender. Drain and peel as soon as they are cool enough to handle – it is easier to remove the skin when the potatoes are hot. Purée them using a food mill or potato ricer directly onto the work surface.

Purée the beetroots straight on top of the potato mound. Mix the two purées together and gradually add the flour, while kneading the mixture. Stop adding flour when you have a soft, elastic dough which sticks together. Shape the dough into a ball, wrap it in clingfilm and put aside to rest for some 30 minutes or so. It is easier to shape the mixture when it is cold.

To make the gnocchi, pinch a small ball of the dough and shape it into a sausage, about 2–3cm/¾–1¼in in diameter, and then cut lengths about 2cm/¾in long. You will need to do this on a floured surface and with floured hands. You can either leave the gnocchi as they are or you can flip them along the prongs of a well-floured fork to make the grooves. The grooves are there not just for decoration; they serve to thin out each gnocco and to provide grooves or holes to catch the sauce.

To make the dressing, heat the butter in a small saucepan together with the sage and garlic. Fry gently until the butter is golden. Set aside while you cook the gnocchi.

Bring a large saucepan of water to the boil and drop the gnocchi in the boiling water in batches, not all in one go as they might stick to each other. (I would cook this quantity of gnocchi in 4 batches.) Stir gently with a wooden spoon and cook until the gnocchi come back to float on the surface. This will take about 1–2 minutes after the water has come back to the boil. Leave for a further 30 seconds and then lift the gnocchi out with a slotted spoon and put them in a warmed oven dish. Pat dry with kitchen paper after each addition, pour a little of the sage and butter dressing over and sprinkle with some Parmesan, and pepper if you like.

When all the gnocchi are cooked, remove and discard the garlic from the remaining dressing and pour it over the gnocchi with the crunchy sage leaves. Serve with more Parmesan on the side.

Broccoli e Broccoletti
Broccoli and Broccoletti

The humble broccoli has travelled from the peasant tables of Puglia to 3-star Michelin restaurants in New York, Paris and London. I am delighted this has happened, even though I find it rather odd. It cannot all be due to the health-giving properties of broccoli, which are formidable: it protects against cancer and skin diseases, it lowers blood pressure and cholesterol, it helps digestion and constipation and more besides.

Broccoli has been eaten in Italy since Roman times, but was shunned by chefs because of its cabbage-smelling association. There are no recipes for broccoli in Artusi or Ada Boni's books a hundred years ago or more, while today most cookery books contain at least one recipe for it. Broccoli is often called *cavolfiore* in southern Italy, which also means cauliflower and this confusion of names between regions is common in Italy.

Buy broccoli with tightly closed florets and green, fresh-looking stems. If the recipe requires only the florets, you can use the stems as follows: peel off the thick outer layer, lightly boil the stems and dress them with olive oil. Broccoli is full of flavour and can be cooked in many ways. My favourite broccoli recipe is Orecchiette with Broccoli, a simple recipe where the chewy orecchiette are cooked in the same pan as the tender broccoli and then sautéed in oil with anchovy fillets, garlic and sometimes a pinch or two of dried chilli.

Broccoletti are the green tops of a variety of turnip which are harvested in the spring or early summer before the florets appear. They are often also called cime di rapa or friarelli. Broccoletti have a sweeter flavour than broccoli, not dissimilar to asparagus. Like asparagus, they must be cooked just right; they should bend gently when you lift them up between your thumb and index finger. Serve them dipped in melted butter and then sprinkled with grated Parmesan or cover them with a glossy layer of the best olive oil.

Broccoletti al Pomodoro
Broccoletti with Tomatoes and Spring Onions

Serves 4

300g/10½oz broccoletti

1 bunch spring onions (scallions)

4 tbsp extra virgin olive oil

12 cherry tomatoes

Sea salt and freshly ground black
   pepper

This recipe takes less than 30 minutes to make. The spring onions add a
subtle oniony flavour which enhances the flavour of the broccoletti.

Cut the broccoletti into 5cm/2in pieces, wash and then blanch them for
3 minutes in boiling water. Drain and dry them with kitchen paper.

Remove the outer leaves and the roots of the spring onions, cut them into
5mm/¼in strips and put them in a frying pan with the oil and a pinch of
salt. Cook gently for 10 minutes, stirring frequently.

Make a cut at the bottom of each tomato, plunge them in boiling water for
20 seconds, drain and peel them. Coarsely chop and add to the onion. Cook
for 10 minutes and then add the broccoletti and salt and pepper to taste.
Cook over a low heat for 15–20 minutes, stirring the broccoletti around in
the sauce every now and then.

Broccoli in Padella con la Pancetta
Sauteed Broccoli with Pancetta

Serves 4

350g/12oz broccoli

3 tbsp olive oil

150g/5½oz smoked pancetta cubes

3 garlic cloves, bruised

Sea salt and freshly ground black
   pepper

In padella means the broccoli is cooked in a pan without first being boiled.
It is a very good method because it preserves the flavour of the broccoli
better. I prefer using smoked pancetta, but unsmoked will do instead.

Separate the broccoli florets from the stems, discard the stems and cut the
larger florets into smaller pieces. Wash and drain the florets.

Heat 1 tbsp of the oil in a sauté pan large enough to hold the florets more
or less in a single layer. When the oil is hot, add the pancetta cubes. Fry
until crisp and then remove them to a side dish using a fish slice.

Add the remaining oil and the garlic to the pan and, after about 1 minute,
add the broccoli florets and continue frying for a further 5 minutes, turning
them over frequently. Pour in 3–4 tbsp of hot water and cover the pan with
a lid. Cook over a low heat for about 10 minutes until the broccoli is tender.
Stir occasionally during the cooking. When the broccoli is cooked, return
the pancetta to the pan, season with pepper and check the salt. Cook for a
minute or two longer and then serve.

Cecamariti
Broccoletti with Pulses

The Italian title of this recipe means 'It blinds the husbands'. The friend from Puglia who cooked it for me said, 'And it should be so hot to be able to do that'. Well, my husband did not get blind by eating it; he actually enjoyed it very much. Maybe I should have included more chilli.

I prefer to use Puy or Castelluccio lentils, but continental lentils are also good cooked in this way.

Serves 6

1 x 200g/7oz carton or can chickpeas

1 x 200g/7oz carton or can cannellini beans

100g/3½oz Puy or Castelluccio lentils

1 bay leaf

125ml/4fl oz/½ cup extra virgin olive oil

1 large red onion, chopped

300g/10½oz cherry tomatoes, peeled, and halved

1 garlic clove, chopped

2–3 tsp chilli (chili) flakes

150g/5½oz shelled fresh peas, cooked or frozen peas, thawed and drained

500g/1lb 2oz broccoletti

Sea salt

Drain and rinse the chickpeas and the cannellini.

Put the lentils in a saucepan and add 250ml/9fl oz of water and the bay leaf. Bring to the boil and cook until tender – about 20 minutes. Strain but keep the liquid.

Heat 4 tbsp of the oil in a large frying pan and, when hot, add the onion, tomatoes, garlic and chilli. Cook over a lively heat for some 10 minutes, breaking the tomatoes with the back of the spoon. Add the chickpeas, cannellini, drained lentils and peas and cook gently for 10 minutes, stirring frequently.

Meanwhile, wash the broccoletti and cook them for 5 minutes in a saucepan full of boiling, salted water. Drain and add to the pan with the pulses mixture. Add 3–4 tbsp of the lentil cooking liquid and then pour in the remaining oil. Mix well, check the salt to taste and serve.

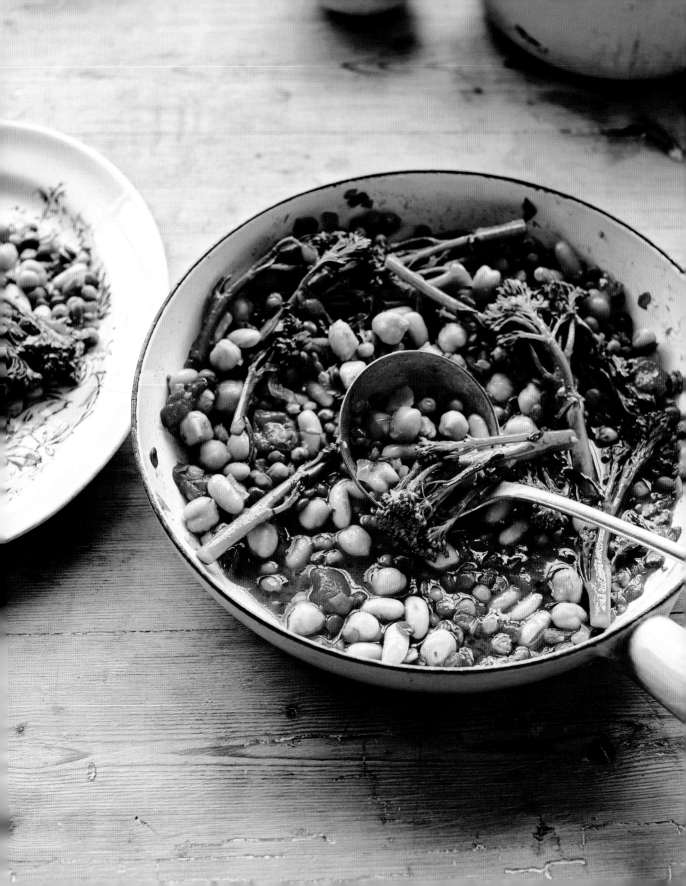

Carciofo
Globe Artichoke

This is for me the most Italian of all vegetables. The artichoke is the emblem of Italy in all its different colours, shapes and sizes, along with the tomato. There are many varieties of artichokes, some with thorns and some without. Artichokes have been eaten around the Mediterranean basin since time immemorial. They became extremely fashionable in the 16th century, thanks to Isabella Gonzaga, who was as keen and knowledgeable on food as she was on art. From Italy the artichoke invaded France and the rest of Europe, arriving in England in the 17th century. However, in Britain artichokes have never been popular, partly because they do not grow well in the climate. The only well known variety here is the big Breton. I am not a fan of this variety, which has limited uses other than being boiled. But in many food markets you can buy the small varieties and here are two recipes using them.

Young artichokes with thorns, called *spinosi*, are usually eaten raw, each leaf dipped in olive oil seasoned with a little salt. Artichokes without thorns are cooked in many different ways, but hardly ever just boiled. When we had a flat in Venice, one of my favourite daily jaunts was shopping at the Rialto market, where I could buy *canarino* artichokes, a small, yellow variety (hence the name meaning 'canary bird'). I would cook them either *alla Giudea*, a recipe from the Jewish ghetto of Rome, or *alla Sarda*, as in the recipe on page 28. Artichokes can also be stuffed with prosciutto, breadcrumbs and cheese and baked.

To prepare artichokes, the tough outer leaves and the hairy 'beard' or 'choke' near the heart of older artichokes need to be removed before cooking. First fill a bowl with cold water and add a few slices of lemon – as soon as you cut the artichoke you need to add it to this water to prevent it from discolouring. Cut off the stalks, peel off their outer layer and discard. Cut the marrow inside the stalks into 3–4cm/1¼–1½in pieces and add to the acidulated water. Now hold the artichoke with one hand and with the other break off the tough outer leaves and discard until you get to the tender leaves. Bend each leaf back with a sharp movement and break off the green top. Continue snapping off the green tops until you get to the central cone of paler leaves with a purplish-green top. Now cut about 1cm/½in off the top of the cone and throw the cleaned artichoke into the acidulated water.

Carciofi coi Piselli
Artichokes and Peas

Artichokes and peas cooked together as in this recipe are a perfect match. The sweetness of the peas seems to enhance the earthy flavour of the artichoke and the result is pure heaven.

If you buy fresh peas in their pods you will need at least 500g/1lb 2oz. Try to buy small artichokes, not the big Breton variety.

Serves 4

6 small artichokes

3 tbsp olive oil

15g/¹/₂oz/1 tbsp unsalted butter

2 banana shallots, chopped

150ml/5fl oz/²/₃ cup vegetable stock

300g/10¹/₂oz shelled fresh peas or frozen peas, thawed and drained

15g/¹/₂oz/scant 1 cup marjoram leaves, chopped

Sea salt and freshly ground black pepper

Prepare the artichokes following the instructions on page 26. Take the cleaned artichokes and cut in half. Remove the fuzzy part attached to the 'heart' and cut each half in segments about 2cm/¾in thick. Put the segments back in the acidulated water while you cook the *soffritto*.

Heat the oil and butter in a large sauté pan. Throw in the shallots and a pinch or two of salt and sauté gently for some 7–8 minutes, stirring frequently. Drain the artichokes and add to the pan. Fry gently for 10 minutes. Add the stock and peas and cook until they are done to your liking.

Sprinkle the marjoram leaves over the artichokes, season with salt and pepper and serve.

Carciofi alla Sarda
Baked Artichokes with Herbs

Artichokes abound in Sardinia, where this recipe comes from. Due to the mild climate of the island they are in the market from October until May. There are many different varieties: with thorns, without thorns, green, yellow, purplish, fat, slim – all sorts.

I came across this dish in a hotel tucked away in an isolated spot of extreme beauty in the mountains of central Sardinia. The landscape may have been rugged and wild but the hotel most certainly was not. It was first class and served food worthy of a Michelin star. Roasted piglets – a local speciality – hang around a huge fireplace, while in another room you could enjoy a vast array of local pecorino cheeses, from mild and sweet ones to very strong, aged cheeses, accompanied by a glass of chilled Verdicchio, the local white wine.

Try to buy small artichokes, not the big Breton variety.

Serves 4

8 small artichokes

2 waxy potatoes, peeled and cut into chunks

15–25g/½–1oz/1 cup flat leaf parsley

10 mint leaves

12 blades of chive

2 garlic cloves

A grating of nutmeg

Sea salt and freshly ground black pepper

125ml/4fl oz/½ cup extra virgin olive oil

Heat the oven to 160°C Fan/180°C/350°F/Gas Mark 4.

An earthenware or cast iron pot is best for this dish as it can be put straight on the heat. It should be large enough to hold all the artichokes standing up in a single layer.

Prepare the artichokes following the instructions on page 26. Put the artichokes and the artichoke stalks in the dish interspacing them here and there with the potatoes. Pour in enough water to come halfway up around the artichokes.

Chop together the parsley, mint, chives and garlic. Put the mixture in a bowl and add a generous grinding of nutmeg, pepper and some salt. Mix in the oil and then pour over the artichokes. Put the dish on a high heat and bring to the boil.

Cover the dish and place it in the oven for 30–40 minutes, until the point of a knife enters easily into the bottom of the artichokes. If there is still too much liquid when the artichokes are done, lift the artichokes out of the pot and put to one side. Reduce the liquid over a high heat. Taste and check the seasoning in the juices and then place 2 artichokes on each plate and pour some of the juices, artichoke stalks and potato pieces over. Serve warm or at room temperature.

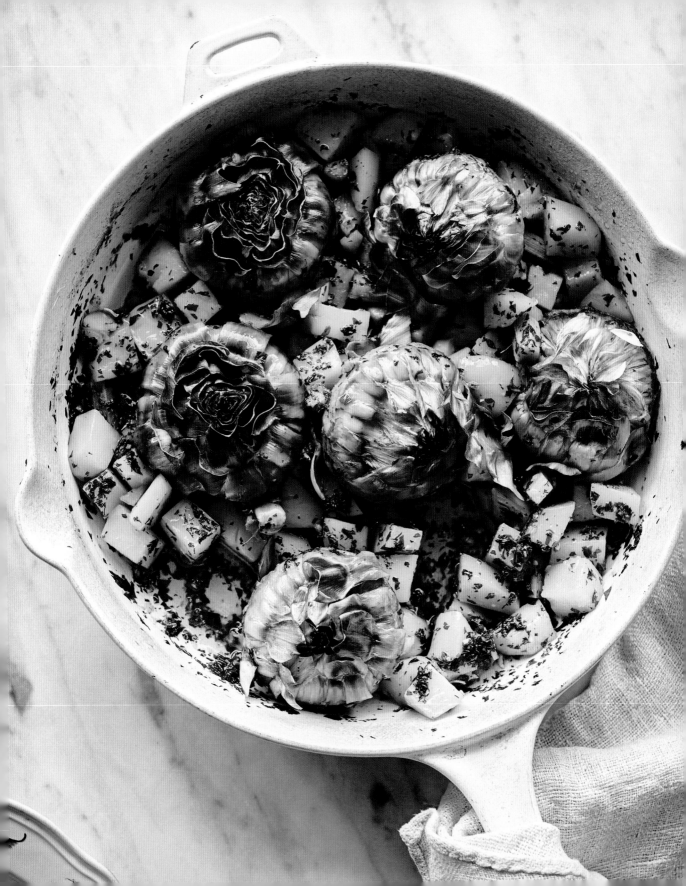

Cardo
Cardoon

The cardoon is a spectacular Mediterranean thistle, like the globe artichoke, but with cardoons it is the stem that is eaten, not the flower bud. In its method of cultivation it is more akin to celery than to artichoke, but its flavour is reminiscent of the artichoke, though slightly sweeter. In central Italy it is also called *gobbo* (hunchback) because of the way the plant curves during blanching.

When young, cardoons are eaten raw, as they are with the Piedmontese dish, *Bagna Caôda* (see below), to which they are the main accompaniment. They can also be cooked in very little water, flavoured with oil, garlic and parsley and finished off with a light sauce of egg yolk and lemon.

Only the inner stalks and the heart of older cardoons are eaten. When cut they should be rubbed with lemon to prevent discoloration and then simmered in water for 30–45 minutes, after which they may be dressed with anchovy butter, or baked in the oven with butter and grated Parmesan, or served with béchamel sauce.

Bagna Caôda
Hot Garlic and Anchovy Dip for Raw Vegetables

Serves 6–8
50g/1 ¾oz/4 tbsp unsalted butter
4 garlic cloves, very finely sliced
5 salted anchovies, boned and rinsed, or 10 canned or bottled anchovy fillets, drained
200ml/7fl oz/generous ¾ cup extra virgin olive oil, preferably Ligurian or another mild variety

Bagna caôda is a popular Piedmontese antipasti. The name means 'hot bath', since this sauce is kept hot when it's at the table, usually in an earthenware pot over a spirit flame. The vegetables for dipping into it can be anything seasonal. Traditional choices include raw peppers, cardoons, cabbage, celery and fennel. Then, when there is only a little of the sauce left, eggs are broken into it and scrambled. It is a very old sauce, already popular in the 16th century and then, as now, is a convivial dish for festive occasions, shared by everyone at the table.

Melt the butter in a small, deep, earthenware pot or a very heavy-bottomed saucepan over the lowest possible heat. As soon as the butter has melted, add the garlic and sauté for a few seconds. The garlic should not colour.

Add the anchovies to the pot and pour in the olive oil very gradually, stirring the whole time. Cook for about 10 minutes, always on the lowest possible heat and stirring constantly until the ingredients are well blended.

Bagna Caôda: See image on page 6

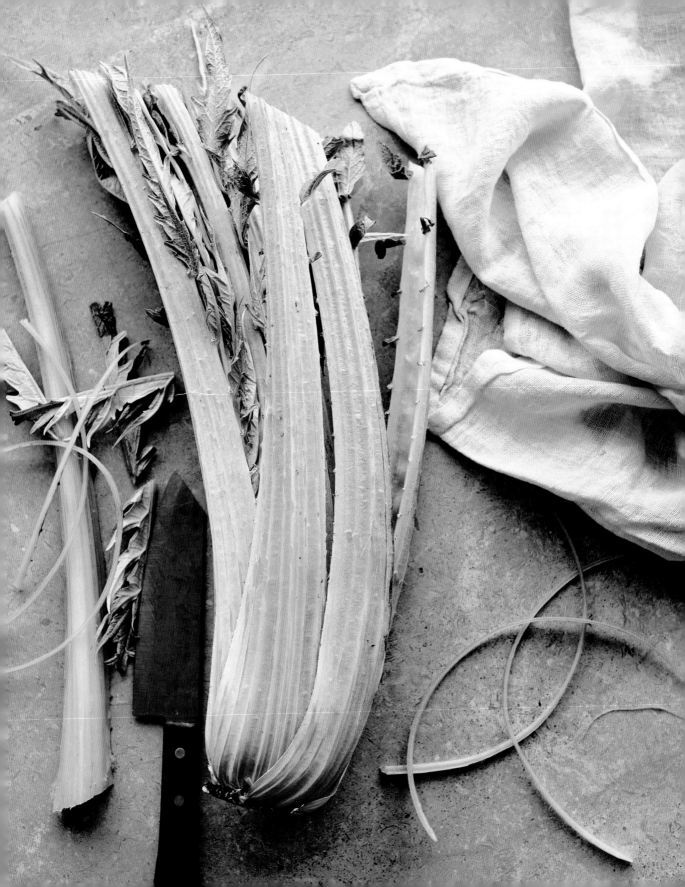

Carota
Carrot

Carrots have been eaten in Italy since Roman times. They have always been popular, probably more in northern Italy than in the south. In my home in Milan they were often served as a *contorno* (an accompaniment) – to *saltimbocca* or veal *cotolette*. And the recipe here is a real classic.

There are many different varieties of carrots, which come in a range of different colours, from ivory to purplish pink, but the most common is the orange carrot, and their taste is the same. Buy slim carrots, but not the baby ones, which have not yet developed any flavour. If they have a top, see that it is green. I am not in favour of serving carrots with their green tops still on, however pretty this looks; a lot of earth still lurks in between the fronds and you will find bits of grit under your teeth.

Carrots are one of the vegetables used in a *battuto*, a finely chopped or 'beaten' vegetable and herb mixture which is the point of departure of many Italian dishes; carrot gives the *battuto* a touch of sweetness which is often, if not necessary, at least very welcome.

Carrots are also used in soups, stocks, marinades or eaten raw, usually grated and dressed with olive oil and lemon juice. I make a sauce with grated carrot to serve with roast or boiled meats: sauté grated carrots and chopped onion together in some olive oil and butter; then add vinegar, tomato purée, stock and sugar to the mixture and cook for about 30 minutes.

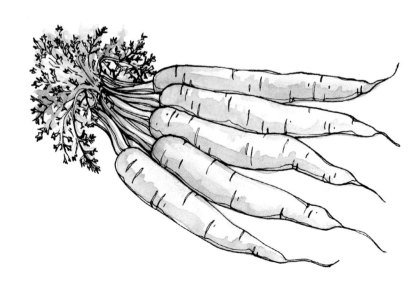

Carote in Agrodolce
Carrots in Sweet and Sour Sauce

Serves 6

6 tbsp olive oil

1 garlic clove, chopped

25g/1oz/1 cup flat leaf parsley, chopped

6 mint leaves, chopped

1kg/2lb 4oz carrots, very thinly sliced into discs

3 tbsp balsamic vinegar

½ tbsp brown sugar

Sea salt and freshly ground black pepper

Agrodolce is a sweet and sour sauce made with wine vinegar and sugar as its base and many vegetables are cooked this way. Carrots work particularly well, as the vinegar brings out the intrinsic sweetness of the vegetable. I used to cook the carrots directly on the heat, but I now prefer the oven method used here. This dish is delicious eaten straight away, but possibly is even better served cold as an antipasto.

Heat the oven to 180°C Fan/200°C/400°F/Gas Mark 6.

Take a large cast iron casserole dish and pour in the oil. Add the garlic and half the herbs and cook gently until the garlic is fragrant. Add the carrots and stir thoroughly so that they become flavoured with the garlicky oil. Cook for 2 minutes and then add the balsamic vinegar, sugar, salt and a good deal of pepper and continue cooking for about 3 minutes, stirring gently the whole time.

Cover the dish and place in the oven for 30 minutes. About halfway through the cooking, mix in about 2 tbsp of boiling water. At the end of the cooking the carrots will still be quite crunchy and will have absorbed most of the liquid. Taste and adjust the salt and sprinkle over the remaining herbs.

Carote Saltate
Carrots Sautéed in Butter

Serves 4

500g/1lb 2oz carrots, sliced into 3mm/⅛in discs and dried

25g/1oz/1½ tbsp unsalted butter

2 tbsp olive oil

1 small onion, very finely chopped

1 tbsp flour

1 tsp sugar

200ml/7fl oz/scant 1 cup vegetable stock or water

Sea salt and freshly ground black pepper

This is the classic recipe for carrots *all'italiana* as used in my home in Milan, with the difference that now I use a little olive oil as well as butter.

Heat the butter and the oil in a sauté pan and add the onion. Cook over a moderate heat for 5 minutes, turning the onion mixture.

Add the carrots to the onion and continue cooking for 5 minutes on a moderate high heat. Sprinkle with the flour and sugar, stir for 1 minute and then season with salt and add a little stock or water. Do not add all the liquid at once – just gradually whenever necessary during the cooking. Turn the heat down and cook until the carrots are done, which will take about 30 minutes. Don't forget to stir them every now and then and add some of the stock or water if they catch on the bottom of the pan. If you like, season with freshly ground pepper before serving.

Carote alla Siciliana
Carrots Braised in Marsala

Serves 4

50g/1³/₄oz/4 tbsp unsalted butter
750g/1lb 10oz carrots, sliced
125ml/4fl oz/¹/₂ cup Marsala or sherry
*   (but not dry)*
1 tbsp flour
100ml/3¹/₂fl oz/scant ¹/₂ cup vegetable
*   stock*
Sea salt and freshly ground black
*   pepper*

Carrots are not a Sicilian vegetable and seldom appear on local restaurant menus. But like every other vegetable, they grow well in the fertile volcanic soil of that heavenly island. I first had this dish at a dinner party given by Giuseppe di San Giuliano in late September in his splendid garden near Siracusa. With some roasted potatoes, they were the *contorno* or accompaniment to roasted wild rabbit shot on the estate. It was an unforgettable dinner both for the food and for the surroundings.

Melt the butter in a large sauté pan and, when the foam begins to subside, add the carrots, a handful at a time, so that each addition can be stirred properly into the butter. Add the Marsala or sherry and cook over a high heat for 1 minute before sprinkling in the flour.

Cook, stirring constantly for a further minute and then pour in half the stock. Season with salt and pepper, cover the pan and cook, over a low heat, until the carrots are tender – about 20 minutes. Keep a watch on the pan and add a little more stock if the carrots begin to stick to the bottom. Taste and adjust the seasoning before serving.

Vellutata di Carote
Carrot Soup

Serves 2–4

25g/1oz/1¹/₂ tbsp unsalted butter
2 tbsp olive oil
1 large shallot, chopped
500g/1lb 2oz carrots, cut into 1cm/
*   ¹/₂in discs*
5mm/¹/₄in piece root ginger
600ml/20fl oz/2¹/₂ cups vegetable stock
Sea salt and freshly ground black
*   pepper*

This is a smooth soup, excellent served either hot or cold. It is also quick and easy to make.

Heat the butter and oil in a saucepan and when the butter is turning brown, add the shallot and 2 pinches of salt and sauté gently over a very low heat for about 7 minutes, stirring frequently. The shallot should soften and not become golden.

Now add the carrots and grate the ginger into the pan. Mix again and cook for 5–6 minutes, turning the carrots over and over. Add the stock and bring to the boil. Simmer gently for about 25 minutes, until the carrots are soft.

Then purée the soup. I use a stick blender which is by far the easiest method. A liquidizer gives a smoother result. Taste and adjust the seasoning if necessary, and serve hot.

Right: Carote alla Siciliana

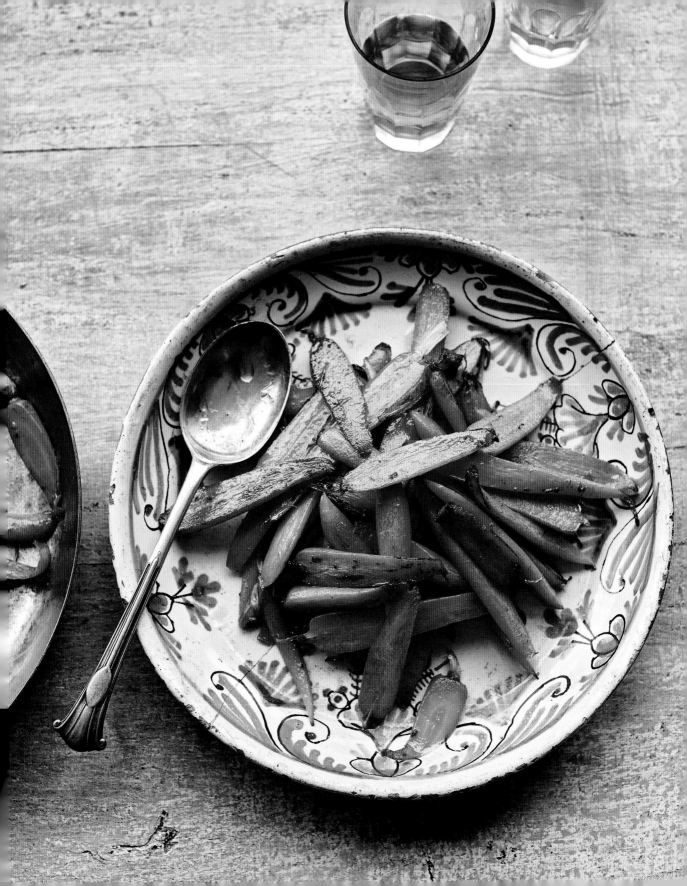

Insalata di Carote, Sedano di Verona e Noci
Carrot, Celeriac and Walnut Salad

This is a salad from northern Italy where celeriac is a well-known vegetable, while it is nearly unknown in the south of the country.

You need approximately half a medium-size celeriac for this salad. Try to buy one with compact roots which will be easy to cut out. I give the weight of the cleaned celeriac – i.e. when the roots have been cut off – simply because some roots have a lot of waste.

When you buy walnut kernels, buy as fresh as possible, as when they are old they have a very unpleasant flavour. Take a good peep inside the packet, if you can – the kernels should appear whole and unblemished. If they are broken up and powdery, forget them.

Serves 4 as a side dish
250g/9oz young carrots
250g/9oz celeriac, cleaned
Juice of ½ unwaxed lemon
4 tbsp olive oil
2 tsp Dijon mustard
1 tbsp wine vinegar
1 tbsp balsamic vinegar
*Sea salt and freshly ground black
    pepper*
*50g/1¾oz/scant ¼ cup walnut kernels,
    coarsely chopped*

Scrub and wash the carrots. Grate them with the grating disc of a food processor or on the large holes of a cheese grater. Put the carrot in a bowl. Do the same with the cleaned celeriac and add to the carrots. Add the lemon juice and a pinch or two of salt and stir well.

Pour the oil into a small bowl, beat in the mustard and the two vinegars. Season with salt and pepper and mix again. Spoon the dressing over the salad and mix the whole thing together very thoroughly. Taste and add salt if necessary.

Sprinkle the walnuts on top of the salad before serving.

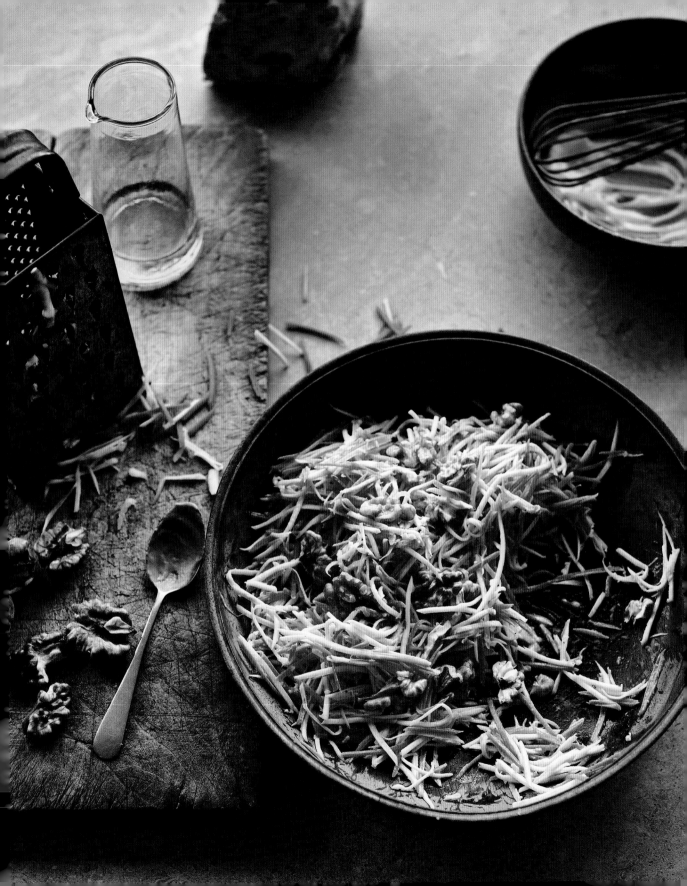

Cavolfiore
Cauliflower

Cauliflower is a vegetable of the cabbage family in which the florets have stopped developing. It can vary in size and colour, which can range from purple to ivory, the most common variety. The flavour, however, remains unchanged. In southern Italy broccoli is often called *cavolfiore*, which can be confusing.

Cauliflower has always been a popular vegetable in Italy. It can be eaten raw, when the florets are young, or cooked in many different ways. Cauliflower cheese or *cavolfiore al gratin* is popular in northern Italy; pasta sauces can be made with the small florets and cauliflower can be braised in both tomato and meat sauces – in a word, it is a very versatile vegetable. I love it blanched and simply dressed with olive oil and lemon juice with, maybe, a few anchovy fillets and some capers thrown in for good measure. But, as Bartolomeo Scappi, the famous 16th-century Italian chef and cookery book author, advised, do not overcook it or it loses so much of its flavour.

To prepare, remove the coarse, outer leaves and cut out some of the central stalk and discard You can always use the leaves in a soup. You can use the tender, pale green leaves around the cauliflower head in the recipes. Most recipes require the head cut into small florets before cooking.

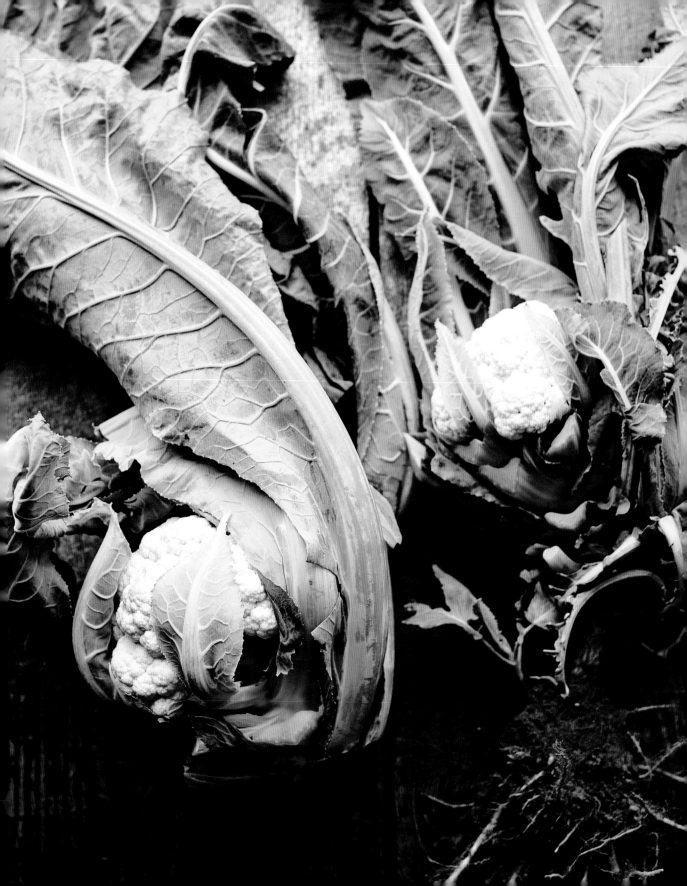

Insalata di Rinforzo
Cauliflower Salad with Anchovies

Serves 4

1 cauliflower, coarse outer leaves and
    central stalk removed

50g/1¾oz stoned (pitted) black olives

50g/1¾oz stoned (pitted) green olives

50g/1¾oz gherkins

1 jar red pepper preserved in vinegar,
    cut into strips

2 tbsp capers

8 anchovy fillets, drained

1 garlic clove

4 tbsp extra virgin olive oil

2 tbsp wine vinegar

Sea salt and freshly ground black
    pepper

This salad is traditionally eaten on Christmas Eve in Naples, Christmas Eve being a meatless day for the Catholic Church. Nowadays few people observe these rules, but some dishes are still traditionally made and eaten on certain days. Personally, I don't want to wait until Christmas Eve for my *cavolfiore di rinforzo* as I like to eat it any day of the year.

Cut the head of the cauliflower in quarters. Cook the stalks, tender, pale green leaves and the head in boiling, salted water for about 7–8 minutes until tender. Drain and cut the stalks and leaves into small pieces and the head into small florets. Add to the serving bowl. Mix in the olives, gherkins, red pepper and capers.

Coarsely chop the anchovy fillets and the garlic together and add to the salad. Mix in the olive oil and vinegar and season with salt and a generous grinding of pepper. Toss well, using two forks, which are better tools than spoons for separating all the bits of salad.

Cavolfiore alla Paesana
Cauliflower and Potatoes Braised in Tomato Sauce

Serves 4

1 cauliflower, about 700g/1lb 9oz,
    coarse outer leaves and central stalk
    removed

6 new potatoes

6 tbsp olive oil

1 onion, finely chopped

2 garlic cloves, finely chopped

12 small fresh plum tomatoes, peeled
    and halved

1 tbsp tomato purée (paste)

2 sprigs of fresh thyme

Sea salt and freshly ground black
    pepper

In Italy vegetables are very often cooked with tomatoes. This dish is especially good eaten on its own so that you can do justice to it

Cut the cauliflower head into small florets, wash and drain them. Scrub the potatoes and cut them in half.

Heat the oil in a saucepan, add the onion and garlic and a generous pinch of salt and sauté for about 5 minutes, stirring very frequently. When the onion is golden, add the potatoes, mix well and after about 2 minutes add the cauliflower. Sauté for 3–4 minutes, turning the vegetables frequently. Add the tomatoes, tomato purée and sprigs of thyme and continue cooking the mixture for a further 2 minutes, stirring the whole time.

Pour in about 150ml/5fl oz/⅔ cup of hot water, season with salt and pepper and bring to the boil. Cover with a lid and cook over a low heat for about 30 minutes until the potatoes and cauliflower are tender. Taste and check the seasoning before serving.

Right: Insalata di Rinforzo

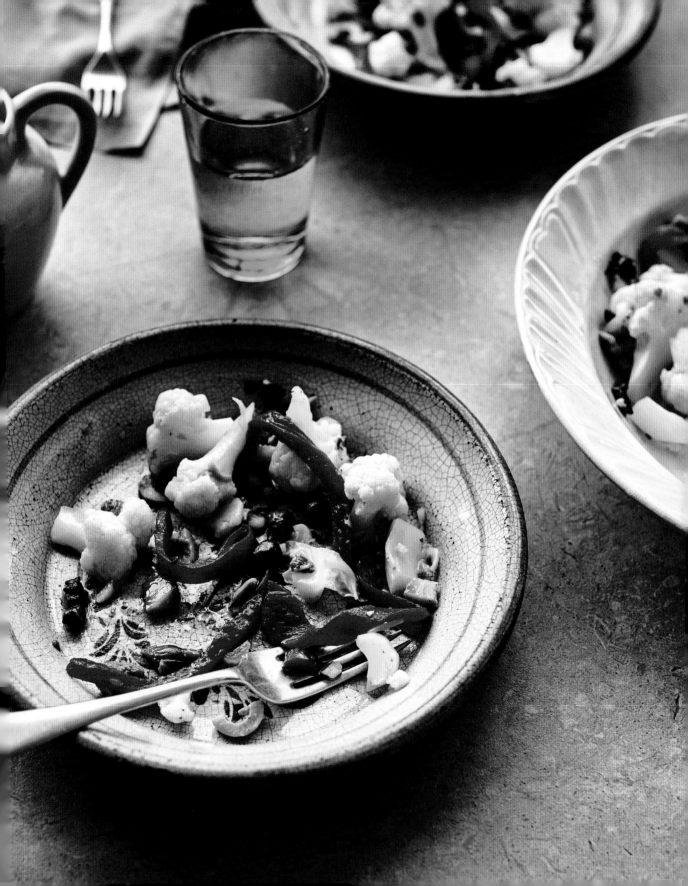

Cavolfiore Ubriaco
Cauliflower Stewed in Wine, or Tipsy Cauliflower

Cauliflower is one of several vegetables I love to cook in wine. Red cabbage (see page 50) and fennel (see page 87) are others.

Serves 4

1 cauliflower, about 700g/1lb 9oz, coarse outer leaves and central stalk removed

25g/1oz/1 cup flat leaf parsley

1 garlic clove

5 tbsp olive oil

½ tsp chilli (chili) flakes

150ml/5 fl oz/²/₃ cup dry white wine

Sea salt

Cut the cauliflower head into quarters. Cut the florets into small pieces and wash and drain them.

Remove the tough stalks from the parsley and chop it together with the garlic. Pour the oil into a sauté pan, add 2 tbsp of the parsley and garlic mixture and the chilli and cook gently until the garlic is fragrant. Mix in the florets and sauté gently for 3–4 minutes, turning the florets over and over to coat in the oil. Add enough boiling water to come about 2cm/¾in up the side of the pan, cover with a lid and cook for 5 minutes.

Pour in the wine and cook, uncovered, and slowly, until the cauliflower is tender, which will take some 20 minutes. It is difficult to be specific about the time as it depends on how fresh the cauliflower is, the size of the florets and also whether you like your cauliflower crunchy or soft. You might have to add a little hot water during the cooking; just keep an eye on it.

When it is cooked to your liking, taste and adjust the salt. You shouldn't need to add any pepper as the chilli should give the dish the right amount of piquancy.

Cavolfiore con la Mollica
Cauliflower with Sautéed Breadcrumbs

In this recipe from Calabria, the cauliflower is served generously sprinkled with breadcrumbs. Breadcrumbs were used in southern Italy instead of grated Parmesan cheese, which was too expensive for the peasants to sprinkle on such a modest dish. Personally, I much prefer cauliflower sprinkled with fried breadcrumbs, especially when they are flavoured with anchovy fillets, as they are in this recipe.

Serves 4

1 small cauliflower, about 500g/
   1lb 2oz, coarse outer leaves and
   central stalk removed
1 garlic clove
4 anchovy fillets, drained
6 tbsp olive oil
½ tsp chilli (chili) flakes
2 tbsp dried breadcrumbs
Sea salt

Cut the cauliflower head into quarters. Cut the florets into small pieces and wash and drain them.

Bring a saucepan of water to the boil, add the cauliflower and season with 1 tbsp of salt. Bring back to the boil and and cook for 3 minutes. Drain the cauliflower.

Cut the garlic in half, remove the germ, if present, and chop together with the anchovy fillets. Transfer the mixture to a frying pan and add 4 tbsp of the oil and the chilli flakes. Fry gently for 1 minute and then add the cauliflower and cook for 5 minutes, turning the cauliflower over and over to coat in the anchovy oil. Check for seasoning and adjust.

Heat the remaining oil in a smaller frying pan and when hot add the breadcrumbs. Cook over a lively heat until all the breadcrumbs are golden and crisp. Transfer the cauliflower to a serving dish, sprinkle the breadcrumbs on top and serve.

Cavolfiore e Piselli al Gratin
Cauliflower and Pea Bake

My mother used to make this dish at home in Milan especially for me. Not really 'especially for me', but with me in mind, since the only vegetables I liked then were peas. So I ate the cauliflower because of the peas. It is an excellent dish which gives a new dimension to everyday cauliflower cheese.

Serves 4

1 medium cauliflower, about 750g/1lb
    10oz, coarse outer leaves and
    central stalk removed
200g/7oz shelled fresh peas or frozen
    peas, thawed and drained
Small knob of butter for greasing the
    dish and for the top
2 tbsp dried breadcrumbs

For the béchamel sauce

500ml/18fl oz/2 cups full-fat (whole)
    milk
50g/1¾oz/4 tbsp unsalted butter
40g/1½oz/¼ cup flour
5 tbsp freshly grated Parmesan
A grating of nutmeg
Sea salt and freshly ground pepper

Cut the cauliflower head into quarters. Cut the florets into small pieces and the more tender stalks into 5–7cm/2–2¾in chunks and wash and drain them.

Heat a saucepan of water and when the water comes up to the boil add 1 tbsp of salt and the stalks of the cauliflower. Boil for 2 minutes and then add the florets. Cook for 5 minutes. If you are using fresh peas, add them to the saucepan about 2 minutes after the florets. If you are using frozen peas, add them to the vegetables at the end of the cooking time. Drain all the vegetables together and set them aside.

Heat the oven to 170°C Fan/190°C/375°F/Gas Mark 5.

The béchamel should be quite a thin sauce. This is how I make it so that it doesn't get lumpy. Heat the milk in a deep saucepan until just beginning to boil. Meanwhile, melt the butter in a small pan on a low heat, add the flour, beating it into the butter for about 1 minute. Then add the hot milk, gradually, while continuing to stir. Stir hard between each addition so it becomes absorbed. When all the milk has been added, place the pan on a heat diffuser and let the sauce simmer gently for 10 minutes, while continuing to stir from time to time. Set aside 1 tbsp of the cheese and add the rest to the sauce, together with the nutmeg, salt and pepper. Mix well, taste and adjust the salt.

Lightly butter an ovenproof dish and add the cauliflower and peas. Spoon the béchamel all over the vegetables. Mix together the remaining grated Parmesan with the breadcrumbs and sprinkle over the top. Dot with the butter and place the dish in the oven. Bake for about 20 minutes until the top has a golden crust. Turn up the temperature a bit if necessary until the crust is golden. Remove from the oven and leave to stand for 2–3 minutes before serving.

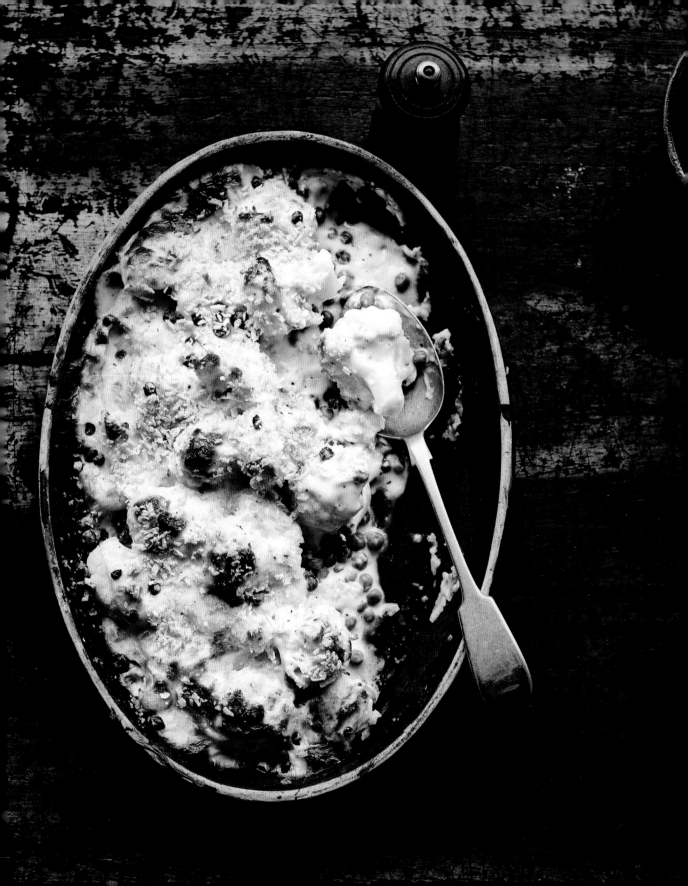

Cavolini di Bruxelles
Brussels Sprouts

Whenever I have a plateful of Brussels sprouts in front of me, I still see myself as a little girl at our dining room table in Via Gesu' in Milan, pushing three or four sprouts around my plate in the hope that they would disappear so that I wouldn't have to eat them. The *cotoletta alla milanese* was happily devoured in a few seconds and so was the potato purée, but the sprouts... And I knew that I had to eat them or they would appear again, first course, at the next meal. They were small and bright green, speckled with golden spots suggesting the gentle sautéeing in butter. Luckily for me, they were not eaten at home very often, as is still the case in most Italian homes today.

Brussels sprouts were not popular in Europe until the late 17th century. Then they began to creep onto English tables and they are now one of the most cherished winter vegetables. Brussels sprouts should be small and tight and then they lend themselves to be braised without being blanched. I sometimes like to braise them in a tomato sauce or in a meat gravy and then they are delicious.

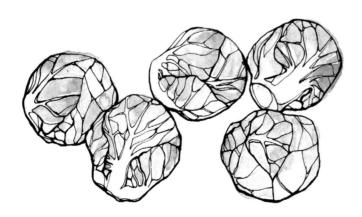

I Cavolini di Bruxelles di Nigella
Roasted Brussels Sprouts with Rosemary, Lemon and Pecorino

This recipe comes from *Nigellissima* (2012), Nigella Lawson's book based on Italian recipes. It is a very interesting book, as well as being excellent. Basically, Nigella takes an Italian dish and she then slightly adapts it to the English taste or 'Britalian' food, as she and I have christened it. And very often the result is better than the original.

The flavour of the sprouts is stronger thanks to the vegetables being roasted in the oven, rather than being sautéed in the pan as is done in Italy. Try, and you'll see what I mean. This is the exact replica of Nigella's recipe. Make sure you use a good-quality flavoured oil.

Serves 4–6

2 tbsp garlic oil

1 tsp finely chopped fresh rosemary needles

Rind of 1 unwaxed lemon, juice optional

500g/1lb 2oz smallish Brussels sprouts, trimmed and halved

2 tbsp grated pecorino or Parmesan

Sea salt and freshly ground black pepper

Preheat the oven to 200°C Fan/220°C/425°F/Gas Mark 7.

Put the garlic oil in a shallow roasting pan, add the rosemary and finely grated lemon rind, and then tumble in the halved sprouts and smoosh everything about in the pan to coat the sprouts as best as you can. Put the pan in the oven and cook for 20 minutes.

Taste to check that the sprouts are cooked through, though a bit of resistance (for this vegetable, in particular) is not a bad thing, and roast them for another 4–5 minutes if necessary; then remove the pan from the oven.

Decant the sprouts into a warmed serving bowl, sprinkle with the cheese, then toss to combine well before adding salt and pepper to taste. If you want to add some lemon juice from the lemon you zested earlier, do.

Cavolini di Bruxelles al Gratin
Brussels Sprouts Bake

This is a delicious way to serve Brussels sprouts. It is really a dish in its own right rather than just being an accompaniment to meat. It is a perfect dish for a vegetarian if you substitute vegetable stock for meat. If you have not got any meat stock, make it with a good meat bouillon.

Serves 4

500g/1lb 2oz Brussels sprouts

50g/1 ¾oz/4 tbsp unsalted butter

1 garlic clove, crushed

1 tbsp flour

150ml/5fl oz/²⁄₃ cup meat or vegetable stock

3 tbsp dried breadcrumbs

4 tbsp freshly grated Parmesan

Sea salt and pepper

Heat the oven to 160°C Fan/180°C/350°F/Gas Mark 4.

Trim and wash the sprouts. Bring a pan of water to the boil and add the sprouts. Cook for 2–3 minutes and then drain.

Heat 30g/1oz of the butter with the garlic and, when the aroma of the garlic rises, throw in the Brussels sprouts. Sauté for 3–4 minutes, turning them over and over so they are coated with butter. Remove the garlic and discard, and put the sprouts in an ovenproof dish.

Set aside a small knob of the butter and heat the remaining butter in a small pan. When the foam begins to subside, mix in the flour, stir rapidly for some 30 seconds and then add the stock, while you continue mixing to incorporate the flour. When the sauce begins to bubble, turn the heat down to a minimum and cook for a further 2–3 minutes, stirring the whole time. Season with salt and pepper. Spoon the sauce over the sprouts.

Mix together the breadcrumbs and Parmesan and sprinkle the mixture over the sprouts. Dot with the last knob of butter, put the dish in the oven and bake for 15–20 minutes. Remove from the oven and set aside to rest for a few minutes before serving.

Cavolo
Cabbage

Cabbage was a favourite vegetable of the Etruscans and the Romans and was widely cultivated, as it is still now in most parts of the peninsula. The three common varieties found in Italy are *cavolo cappuccino*, which includes the types known as primo, white/Dutch (*cavolo bianco*) and red (*cavolo rosso*) and which are suitable for eating raw as well as cooked, *cavolo cinese* which is similar to the *cappuccio* but less compact, and *cavolo verza* or Savoy cabbage which is the most popular. *Cavolo verza* is added to meat dishes, such as *cassoeula* or Milanese pork stew, it is used in soups and is often stuffed, either whole or using the blanched leaves to encase the stuffing. *Cavolo a punta* (pointed cabbage) is also very popular.

Then there is the *cavolo nero* or black cabbage which has a very different appearance from the other varieties. It has elongated, green-bluey leaves with a stalk, which should be partly removed before cooking. It is the most popular cabbage variety in Tuscany where it is one of the basic ingredients for the soup *Ribollita* (see page 56).

What would the British have done without cabbage in the many years leading up to the 1990s? When I arrived in England, it was the usual accompaniment to meat, fish and all, usually overcooked and served as it was without a drop of oil or a lump of butter. I love cabbage when it is perfectly cooked, slightly crackling under your teeth and full of that peculiar brassica flavour which is the delight of cabbage lovers. Rather than boil cabbage, I prefer to cut it into thin strips or finely shred it, then braise it or cook it simply in butter and a little oil.

Cavolo Rosso Ubriaco
Red Cabbage Cooked in Wine, or Tipsy Red Cabbage

Cabbage is often cooked in wine in Trentino and other mountainous areas of northern Italy which were part of the Austro-Hungarian Empire until 1918 – just think of sauerkraut. Instead of red cabbage (*cavolo rosso*), you can use pointed cabbage (*cavolo a punta*) or Savoy cabbage (*cavolo verza*).

Serves 4

1 red cabbage

1 onion

The needles of 2 sprigs of rosemary

2 garlic cloves

2 tbsp olive oil

200ml/7fl oz/generous ¾ cup red or
    white wine, depending on what you
    have available

Sea salt and freshly ground black
    pepper

Cut the cabbage in half, then in quarters and remove the hard core. Cut the quarters into thin shreds, wash and drain them. The easiest way to wash shredded cabbage is to put it in a colander and place the colander in a sink full of water to reach the top of the colander. Give a good swish around and then lift the colander out of the sink.

Chop the onion, rosemary and garlic together. Place the mixture in a large pan and add the oil. Cook for 5 minutes and then add the cabbage, a few handfuls at a time so that it is easier to mix. When all the cabbage has been added, pour in the wine. Add salt and pepper, cover the pan with a lid, and cook over a low heat for about 1 hour. Check that there is enough liquid during the cooking and you might need to add a little boiling water once or twice. When the cabbage is cooked to your own taste, check the seasoning and serve.

Verze Imbracate
Savoy Cabbage Stewed with Sausages

Savoy cabbage or *cavolo verza* is one of the best known vegetables of Lombardy. It grows well there and is cooked in many different ways. Here, it is mixed with *luganega*, the famous Lombardy sausage which you can buy online or in Italian delis. If not, buy the best coarse-grained, pure pork sausages you can find and without any added flavouring.

Serves 4

500g/1lb 2oz Savoy cabbage

500g/1lb 2oz luganega sausage or
   4 pure pork sausages

1 tbsp olive oil

50g/1³⁄₄oz unsmoked pancetta cubes

1 small onion, finely chopped

3 tbsp wine vinegar

Sea salt and freshly ground black
   pepper

Heat the oven to 160°C Fan/180°C/350°F/Gas Mark 4.

Cut the cabbage into thin strips, wash and drain. Cut the sausage or sausages into 3cm/1¼in chunks.

Heat the oil with the pancetta in an ovenproof casserole dish and cook until crisp. Add the onion and a pinch of salt and continue cooking until the onion is soft and translucent. Add the cabbage to the dish, mix well for a minute or two and add the sausages. Pour in the vinegar, season with salt and pepper and cover with a lid. Place in the oven and cook for 40–50 minutes. Check halfway through the cooking to see whether there is enough liquid. If necessary add a little boiling water or stock. Check the seasoning before serving.

Cavolo Saltato
Sautéed Spiced Cabbage

This recipe gives a new, interesting twist to the everyday white cabbage (*cavolo bianco*).

Serves 4

½ white cabbage

1 red onion

1 garlic clove

2 tbsp olive oil

Chilli (chili) flakes to taste

1 tbsp tomato purée (paste)

500ml/18fl oz/2 cups chicken or beef
    stock, either homemade or made
    with bouillon powder or cube

Sea salt and freshly ground black
    pepper

Shred the cabbage very finely – I use a food processor. Put the shredded cabbage in a sink of cold water while you get on with the cooking.

Chop the onion and garlic and place in a sauté pan. Add the oil and a little salt and put the pan on a low heat. Cook gently for 10 minutes, stirring frequently. Drain the cabbage, but do not over drain it, and add to the pan. Mix thoroughly and then add the chilli – I leave it to you how much to add; you might like it hotter than I do.

Dissolve the tomato purée in a little stock and pour into the pan. Mix thoroughly and cook for some 2 minutes and then add about half the remaining stock. Bring to the boil and cook over a low heat for 15–20 minutes, adding a little more stock if the cabbage looks like it's catching on the bottom of the pan. At the end of cooking the cabbage should have absorbed all the liquid. Check the seasoning and serve.

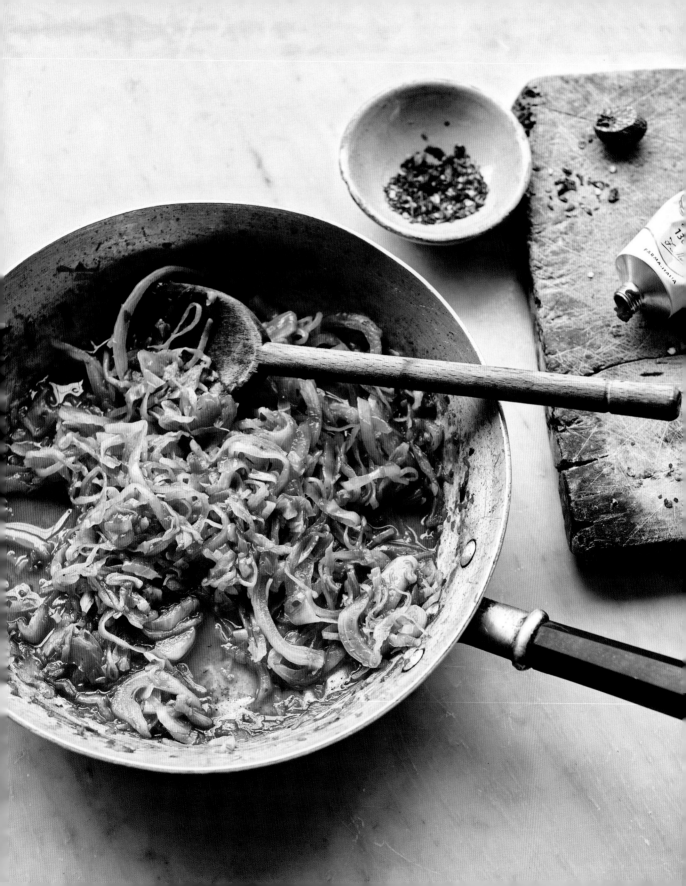

Cavolo Nero e Patate Strascinati
Cavolo Nero and Potatoes Sautéed with Chilli and Garlic

The word *strascinato* means 'dragged'. Here, the *cavolo nero* (as it is often called in English) and potatoes are *strascinati* or dragged around the pan to absorb all the flavours of the oil, chilli and garlic. The potatoes lend substance to the *cavolo nero* and the *cavolo nero* lends its peculiar bitter-cabbagey flavour to the potatoes – a delicious combination.

Serves 4

4 large waxy potatoes, about 750g/
  1lb 10oz
10 leaves of cavolo nero
6 tbsp extra virgin olive oil
2 garlic cloves
2 pinches chilli (chili) flakes
Sea salt

Scrub the potatoes and put them still in their skins in a saucepan. Cover with cold water, add 1 tbsp of salt and cook at a lively simmer until just tender when tested with the point of a small knife. Lift them out of the water with a slotted spoon and place them in a colander until cool enough to peel. Keep the potato water. Peel the potatoes and cut into chunks.

Remove the tougher end of the stalks of the *cavolo nero*, wash the leaves and cut into strips. Bring the potato water back to the boil and then add the *cavolo nero*. Boil until tender, which will take about 15 minutes. Drain well.

While the *cavolo nero* is cooking, heat the oil in a large frying pan and add the garlic and chilli flakes. Sauté until just golden and add the potatoes, mix for a minute or two and then add the *cavolo nero* and continue cooking for 5 minutes or so, turning all the time. Taste and check the salt before serving.

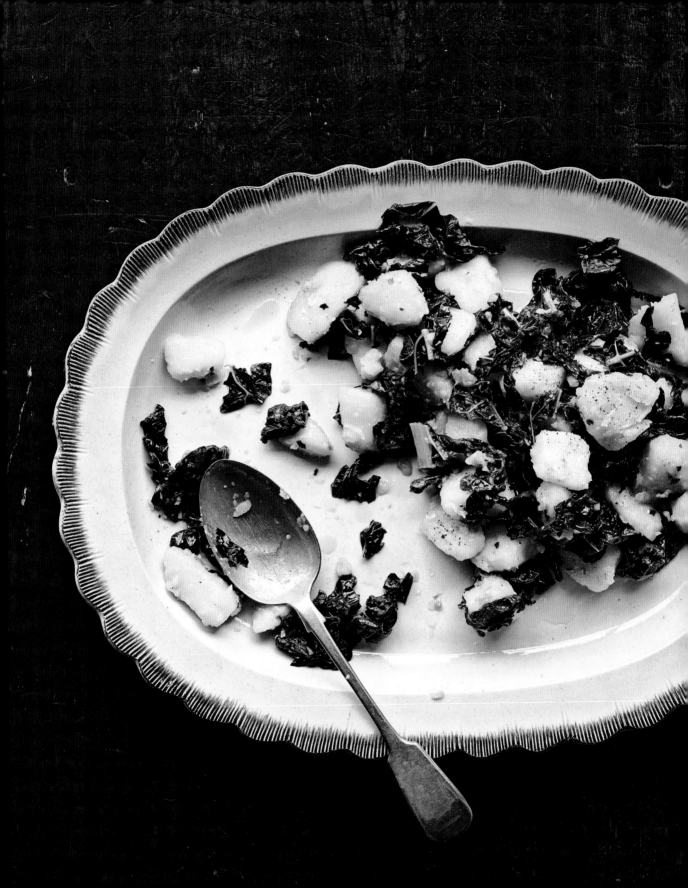

La Ribollita
Tuscan Cavolo Nero Soup

Tuscany is the region of exceptional soups and *La Ribollita* made with *cavolo nero* or black cabbage is the queen of them all. *Ribollita* means 'reboiled', and this soup should be made at least one day in advance and then reboiled before eating. It should be made in an earthenware pot, the sort that can be put directly on the heat and which is well worth having in your kitchen, not only for soups and pulses, but also for stews.

For this soup you should use dried cannellini beans, not the ready to use ones in cans or cartons. This is because you need the liquid in which the beans have been cooked for the stock for the soup.

Serves 8
250g/9oz dried cannellini beans
6 tbsp extra virgin olive oil
2–3 garlic cloves, chopped
The needles of 2 sprigs of rosemary
2 sprigs of thyme
2–3 pinches chilli (chili) flakes
300g/10½oz cavolo nero, large stalk
*   removed and cut into strips*
Sea salt

For cooking the beans
2 tbsp extra virgin olive oil
1 large onion, finely chopped
2–3 garlic cloves, chopped
1 carrot, chopped
1 celery stalk, preferably with leaves,
*   chopped*
1 leek, sliced
3 ripe tomatoes, peeled, seeded and
*   chopped*

First soak the cannellini in cold water overnight or for at least 8 hours. Drain and rinse them under cold water.

To cook the beans, heat the 2 tbsp of oil in a large, earthenware stockpot, add the onion, garlic, carrot, celery, leek and tomatoes and sauté for about 7–8 minutes, turning the vegetables over and over in the oil so they are well coated. This is the *soffritto*.

Add the beans and stir well for 1 minute so that they pick up all the flavours in the *soffritto*. Then add 2 litres/3½ pints/8½ cups of water. Season with salt and cover the pot. Cook, at the gentlest simmer, for at least 2 hours. By then the beans will be very tender. Using a slotted spoon, lift out about half the beans and put them in the bowl of a food processor. Whizz to a purée and then return the purée to the soup. Now the soup is going to rest.

The next day, bring the soup back to the boil, taste and check for salt. While the soup is heating up, pour the oil into a small frying pan. When the oil is hot, throw in the garlic, rosemary, thyme and chilli flakes. Sauté for 1–2 minutes and then add to the soup.

Wash the cavolo nero and add to the soup. Stir well and cook for about 20 minutes until done. And now your *Ribollita* is ready to be enjoyed. Ribollita is usually served without adding cheese on top, but I like to add some grated pecorino.

Zuppa di Cavolo alla Mantovana
Pointed Cabbage and Bread Soup

I love this soup made with pointed cabbage (*cavolo a punto*), but I don't know whether this is for its own sake or for the connection with Mantova (Mantua), a provincial city in Lombardy, which offers some of the best art and food in Italy. Based in Mantova, the Gonzaga dynasty was one of the richest courts in Europe between the 14th and 17th centuries and as such they were able to patronise some of the most famous artists of the time. Frescoes and paintings by Mantegna and Giulio Romano are on show in the Palazzo Gonzaga, which takes up one side of a beautiful, large square.

The other much smaller square is 'home' to the daily market. Last time I was there, it was still a proper food market, with plenty of vegetable, meat, cheese and salami stalls, as well as stalls selling live chicken and rabbit. Unfortunately, the tourist stalls selling belts, bags, pashminas, kimonos and hats are there, too, but I feel that Mantova is still agricultural enough and not touristy enough to keep a good balance between the two.

This is a very thick and nourishing soup, practically a meal in its own right. You can, of course, make this soup with any cabbage.

Serves 4

250g/9oz pointed cabbage

1 tbsp olive oil

50g/1¾oz unsmoked pancetta cubes

1 onion, thinly sliced

½ tbsp tomato purée (paste)

1.5 litres/2½ pints/6½ cups beef stock, homemade or use bouillon powder or cube

4 slices sourdough bread, toasted

2 garlic cloves

Sea salt and freshly ground black pepper

Cut the pointed cabbage into thin strips, wash and drain. Cook for 5 minutes in a saucepan of boiling, salted water, then drain.

Heat the oil in your soup pot, add the pancetta and fry until crisp. Throw in the onion and 2 pinches of salt and cook over a low heat for some 6–8 minutes, stirring frequently so that the onion just softens and becomes golden. Do not let it burn.

Stir in the tomato purée and cook for 30 seconds before adding the cooked cabbage. Stir well so that the cabbage becomes coated in the onion mixture. Pour in the stock. Mix well, cover the pan, bring to the boil, then lower the heat and simmer for 30 minutes. Add salt and pepper, if necessary.

Just before serving, toast the slices of bread, cut the garlic cloves in half and rub each slice with garlic. Put a slice of toast in each of the 4 bowls and ladle the soup on top.

Minestra di Agnello e Verza
Savoy Cabbage and Lamb Soup

Some cooks add pieces of the cooked lamb to the soup before serving and this makes it really nourishing. I prefer it without the lamb because I find the soup quite filling enough.

Serves 4

1 small Savoy cabbage

1–2 tbsp wine vinegar

4 slices wholemeal sourdough bread

2 garlic cloves

50g/1¾oz/4 tbsp grated mature
pecorino

For the stock

1 lamb knuckle

1 onion

1 celery stalk, preferably with leaves,
cut in pieces

2 garlic cloves

1 carrot, cut in half

1 clove

Sea salt and freshly ground black
pepper

First make the stock. Put the lamb knuckle in a stockpot, add the onion, celery, garlic, carrot, clove and salt and pepper and cover with 2 litres/ 3½ pints/8½ cups of cold water. Bring to the boil and cook for 1½–2 hours at a very low simmer. Remove the lamb knuckle and refrigerate it until you come to make the soup. Drain the stock into a bowl. When cold put the bowl in the refrigerator and leave for some hours or overnight. Then, remove all the fat which has solidified at the top. Now your stock is ready to use.

Now make the soup. Discard the coarse, outer leaves of the cabbage, cut the cabbage into quarters and discard the centre of the core. Cut the cabbage into very thin strips. Wash and drain the strips.

Measure the stock. You will need about 1.2 litres/2 pints/5 cups for the soup. If you don't have enough add some water and if you have too much chill the remainder to use on another occasion. Bring the stock to the boil, add the cabbage and the vinegar and cook for about 30 minutes until the cabbage is tender.

If you want to add the lamb meat to the soup, while the soup is cooking, remove the meat from the knuckle and cut it into small pieces. Add to the soup. Mix well, taste and check the seasoning. If you want more acidity to the soup add more vinegar to taste.

Just before serving, toast the slices of bread, cut the garlic cloves in half and rub each slice with garlic. Put a slice of toast in each of the 4 bowls and ladle some soup on top. Sprinkle 1 tbsp of pecorino on top of each bowl and serve with the remaining pecorino on the side.

Ceci
Chickpeas

Chickpeas were appreciated in Roman times and are popular all over Italy, although the best recipes come from the south. There are a number of chickpea and pasta dishes, usually containing tomatoes and garlic and always dressed with olive oil; the pasta varies from region to region, from lagane to ditali and long strands. A salad of chickpeas and rocket is popular in Puglia, and in Rome chickpeas are sautéed in garlic-flavoured oil with rosemary and anchovies, to which a pinch of chilli flakes may be added.

There are two traditional chickpea dishes from the north: *Ceci in zimino*, from Liguria, is a thick soup of chickpeas with spinach and anchovy fillets; *ceci con la tempia*, from Lombardy, is a rich stew of chickpeas, pork ribs and pig's temple – it is traditional fare in Milan on All Souls' Day.

Chickpeas are usually sold dried. Before cooking, they need to be soaked for at least 8 hours, or if they are old ones, for about 12 hours. They are then drained, rinsed and cooked at length. They are also sold in cans, but then they lose some of their delicious mealiness.

Ceci e Pomodori in Padella
Sautéed Chickpeas and Tomatoes

Serves 2

1 x 400g/14oz can chickpeas

6 tbsp extra virgin olive oil

1 garlic clove, finely chopped

1 fresh red chilli (chili), deseeded, cored and cut into thin strips

250g/9oz small fresh plum tomatoes, cut in half

25g/1oz/1 cup marjoram leaves, chopped

A squeeze or two of lemon juice

Sea salt and freshly ground black pepper

These two vegetables are widely cultivated next to each other in the sun-drenched fields of Puglia, the heel of the Italian boot. In this recipe they end together in a pan bathed in olive oil. Using canned chickpeas makes the recipe quick and easy.

Drain and rinse the chickpeas and set aside.

Heat half the oil in a sauté pan, then add the garlic and chilli. Cook for 1 minute and then throw in the tomatoes and stir them in the oil for about 2 minutes. Add the chickpeas, mix well and cook for about 10 minutes, adding a little bit of hot water so that the chickpeas are always cooking in some liquid.

Add the marjoram, lemon juice, salt and a little pepper, if you want, although the piquancy of the chilli should be quite enough. Pour in the remaining oil and mix thoroughly. This dish is equally delicious served warm or at room temperature.

Zuppa di Ceci e Farro
Chickpea and Farro Soup

Farro is the cereal that kept the Roman legions strong: it is, in fact, the precursor of durum wheat. It is extremely nutritious and tastes good, a bit like a mixture between rice and couscous.

In this soup from Tuscany, the farro is cooked in a purée of chickpeas and dressed with olive oil, herbs, garlic and chilli. The result is a peasant soup worthy of a king's table. Dried chickpeas are used, not canned, as the chickpea stock gives the soup the flavour it needs.

The quantities here are for 8–10 people, simply because while you make it, you might as well make it for two meals. It will keep for 2 days in the refrigerator, and is even better reheated. It also freezes well.

Serves 8–10
800g dried chickpeas
2–3 sprigs of sage, stalks and leaves
4–5 sprigs of parsley
2 sprigs of rosemary
3 bay leaves
6 garlic cloves
200g/7oz farro
Sea salt and freshly ground black
*   pepper*

For the soffritto
100ml/3 1/2fl oz/scant 1/2 cup extra
*   virgin olive oil*
2 garlic cloves
The needles of 4 sprigs of rosemary,
*   about 15cm/6in long*
1 tsp chilli (chili) flakes

Soak the chickpeas in cold water for at least 8 hours, then drain and rinse them under cold water. Now they are ready to be cooked.

Put the chickpeas in a large pot and cover them with 2 litres/3½ pints/ 8½ cups of water. Put the herbs in a small piece of muslin and tie into a bundle. Add to the pot, together with the garlic, cover and bring to the boil. Now adjust the lid so that it is slightly askew and reduce the heat so that the soup just simmers. This is quite important when cooking pulses because a real boil would harden them instead of softening. Cook until the chickpeas are done, which can vary from 1½–2 hours.

Remove the bag of herbs and discard. Using a slotted spoon, ladle out about 3 spoonfuls of chickpeas and put them in a bowl. Purée the soup either in the pot with a stick blender – the quickest method – or in a food processor or a blender. Bring the puréed soup back to the boil and add the farro. Season with salt and pepper. Mix well and cook until the farro is tender, which will take at least 20 minutes. When the farro is cooked, return the set aside chickpeas to the pot.

While the farro is cooking, prepare the *soffritto*. Heat the oil in a small frying pan, add the garlic, rosemary needles and chilli and gently cook for about 2 minutes, stirring frequently. You can add more – or less – chilli depending on how you like it. When the garlic is a golden colour, add the *soffritto* to the soup, mix well and turn off the heat.

The Tuscans put a slice of toasted and oiled ciabatta – like a bruschetta – in each bowl before pouring the soup on top. They also put a bottle of their best olive oil on the table for everybody to add a few drops to their soup as a final 'blessing'. An excellent idea.

60

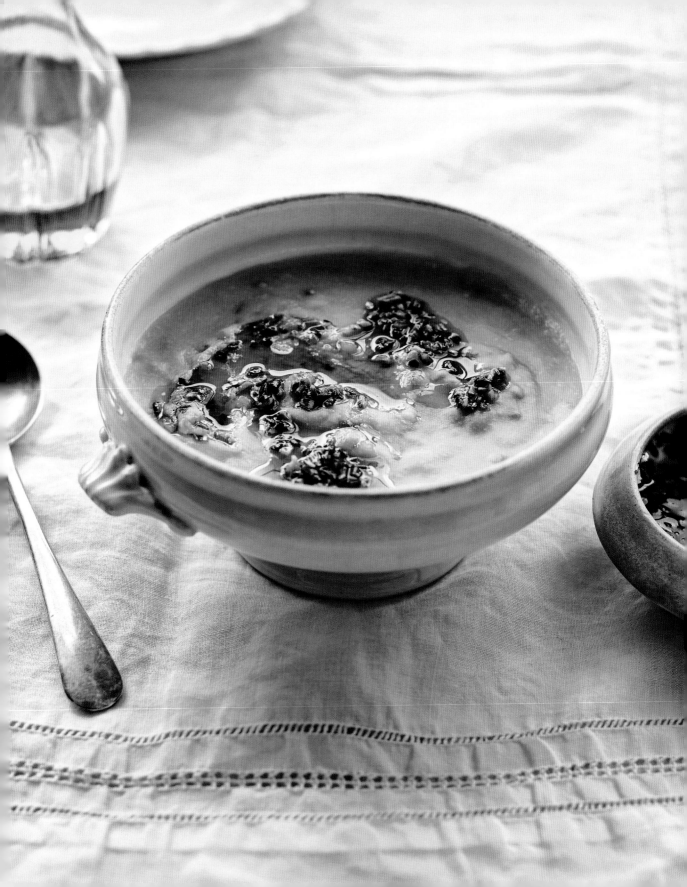

Cetriolo
Cucumber

Italian *cetrioli* are smaller than the English variety. They are also far less popular, eaten only in the summer, usually mixed in a tomato salad with often a few thin slices of red onion. Having said that, I was brought up with 'Insalata di papa', my father's favourite summer salad consisting of thinly sliced cucumber, thinly sliced peppers and sliced tomatoes, dressed only with olive oil, lemon juice and salt. 'No pepper in this salad', he insisted, but I never knew why.

During my long life in England I have become a cucumber addict. It is a very reliable vegetable and can give any salad a welcome crunchiness. I tend to have some always in the drawer of my refrigerator.

L'Insalata del Bronzino
Cucumber, Spring Onion and Purslane Salad

Serves 4

2 small cucumbers

1 bunch spring onions (scallions), foliage and roots discarded

About 25g/1oz purslane, the thickest stalks discarded

4 tbsp extra virgin olive oil

1 tbsp lemon juice

Sea salt and freshly ground black pepper

The recipe here was a favourite of Bronzino, one of the greatest portraitists of the 16th century. I cannot remember where I came across this little poem. I just loved it.

Purslane, which grows wild in many parts of Italy, has fleshy leaves and a rather delicate flavour. It is usually mixed with other vegetables, as in the recipe here, or with herbs like basil or rocket. If you cannot find purslane, substitute with lamb's lettuce.

Un'insalata di cipolla trita
colla porcellanetta e cetrioli
Vince ogni altro piacer di questa vita.

[A salad of chopped onion with purslane and cucumber beats any other pleasure in life.]

Wash and dry the cucumbers. Remove the peel in strips and then slice the cucumbers thinly. Put the slices in a serving bowl and sprinkle with salt. Cut the spring onion bulbs into thin rings. Wash, drain and dry them and add to the bowl. Wash and dry the purslane and add to the bowl.

Pour over the olive oil and lemon juice, add a generous grinding of pepper and toss thoroughly. Taste and add more lemon juice and salt to your liking. I love to add some burrata, 1 ball roughly crumbled on the top. I am sure Bronzino would have approved if he had known burrata.

Cipolla
Onion

Throughout history, onions have been an indispensable ingredient in most cuisines. Apicius was a famous Roman gastronome in the first century AD and many of the recipes he collected use onions mixed with different herbs, sultanas and honey. The Arabs considered onions to be an invigorating food in lovemaking: one writer prescribed a diet of onions and eggs, adhered to for three days, as the best preparation for an 'amorous ordeal'. Many recipes from the Renaissance use onions, at times in combinations that seem odd to our palates. Bartolomeo Scappi, the 16th-century chef and cookery book writer, gives instructions for a sauce of pounded onions, egg yolks, apples and soft breadcrumbs soaked in wine and vinegar. The mixture is then cooked with bitter orange juice, grape juice, sugar and cinnamon, but sadly he does not say which food it should go with.

There are many varieties of onions, from tiny white ones to large specimens of a beautiful purple colour. The onions of Brianza in Lombardy have been appreciated for centuries for their delicate flavour, and for the way they keep their pretty shape all through the cooking. They are often stewed whole in butter and meat stock. The tastiest and mildest onions are grown in Piedmont, where the high mineral content of the soil provides very favourable conditions.

Some recipes call for a particular variety. The red onions of Tropea in Calabria are used in a salad because they are sweet, while the little white ones are ideal in a sweet and sour sauce. Onions are often stuffed, the best-known recipes being from Piedmont. An unusual recipe from the borders of Piedmont and Lombardy mixes Amaretti and Mostarda di Cremona in the stuffing, while another excellent one from Liguria contains preserved tuna. Finely chopped onions are nearly always one of the basic elements of *soffritto*, the starting point for many Italian recipes.

For centuries a typical sight in market towns in northern Italy has been that of people keeping warm on freezing winter mornings by standing near large braziers in which onions are being roasted, with their skins on. The onions are taken home, peeled and sliced, and eaten with olive oil and salt.

Scodelle di Cipolle Ripiene
Onions Stuffed with Tuna

Reviewers and readers usually only notice two or three recipes in any cookery book and I often wonder why some recipes become so successful, while others, equally good, remain unnoticed for ever. One of my most successful was this recipe, first published in *Secrets from an Italian Kitchen* (1989). Because of its success at the time, I felt it needed a new airing and so I have included it in this book.

Serves 4

2–3 large onions, about 500g/1lb 2oz

50g/1¾oz 1-day old sourdough bread, crusts removed

120–150ml/4–5fl oz/½–⅔ cup full fat (whole) milk

200g/7oz best tuna preserved in olive oil

4 anchovy fillets

1 garlic clove

5 tbsp extra virgin olive oil

1 pinch chilli (chili) flakes

1 tbsp capers

2 tsp dried oregano

A squeeze of lemon juice

Dried white breadcrumbs

Sea salt and freshly ground black pepper

Put a large pan of water on the heat and bring to the boil. Wash the onions and put them in the boiling water. Add 1 tbsp of salt and cook for 10–15 minutes, until the onions are just beginning to soften. Drain and set aside.

Break the bread into small pieces, put in a bowl and cover with the milk. Set aside

Drain the tuna and put it in the small bowl of a food processor, together with the anchovy fillets and garlic. Blitz for a few seconds, while adding 1–2 tbsp of the oil through the funnel. Scoop the mixture into a bowl.

Now go back to the onions. Discard the outer skin and cut the onions in half. Gently remove and set aside 16–18 outer leaves. Chop the remaining leaves and put them in a frying pan with 2 tbsp of the oil. Cook over a low heat for 7–8 minutes.

Heat the oven to 180°C Fan/200°C/400°F/Gas Mark 6.

Squeeze the milk out of the bread and add to the onion, together with the chilli, capers and oregano. Mix well and cook for 5 minutes, stirring frequently. Add this mixture to the bowl with the tuna and mix thoroughly. Mix in the lemon juice, taste and add salt, if necessary, although the anchovy fillets and the tuna might be salty enough. Season with a grinding of pepper.

To make the onion cups, place one or two smaller leaves of onion inside a bigger one. When you have made 8 onion cups, fill each cup with some of the stuffing. Brush a baking dish – I use a lasagne dish – with some of the remaining oil and place the onion cups in it, one next to the other. Sprinkle each onion with some dried breadcrumbs, pour the remaining oil over and place the dish in the oven for 20 minutes or until a golden crust has formed on top. Serve warm or at room temperature.

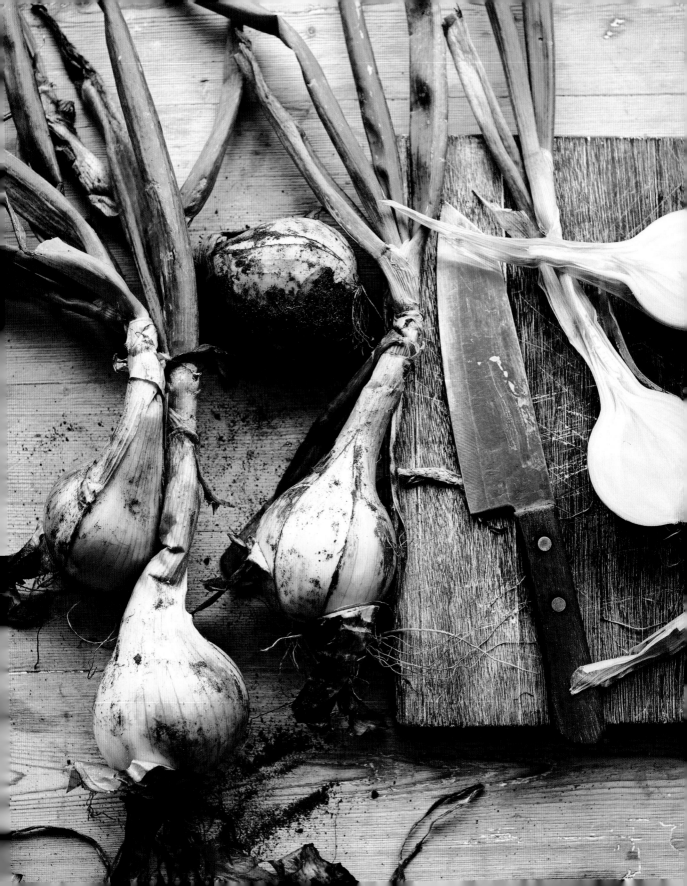

Frittata di Cipolle di Myriam
Baked Onion Frittata

This recipe comes from a dear old friend of mine, Myriam. I first met her over 40 years ago, when she married an Englishman, as I did. We had that in common plus a love for cooking and for eating good food. The exchange of recipes started then and still goes on. I know that I can trust Myriam.

Serves 6–8

2 tbsp olive oil

30g/1oz/2 tbsp unsalted butter

1kg/2lb 4oz onions, very finely sliced

12 eggs

4 tbsp grated Parmesan

Sea salt and freshly ground black pepper

Heat the oven to 160°C Fan/180°C/350°F/Gas Mark 4.

Heat the oil and butter in a large sauté pan. When the foam begins to subside, add the onion, sprinkle with a little salt (this helps the onion to release some liquid and not burn), mix thoroughly and cook gently for about 15 minutes until soft. Stir occasionally until the onion softens and becomes golden.

While the onion is cooking, break the eggs into a bowl and gently beat them. Add a little salt and pepper.

Grease a lasagne dish (25 x 10cm/10 x 4in is ideal) with a little oil. Spoon in the onion with its juices and pour the beaten eggs on top. Bake for 25 minutes and then sprinkle the cheese on top. Put the dish under a hot grill for 2–3 minutes until the top becomes just golden, then serve.

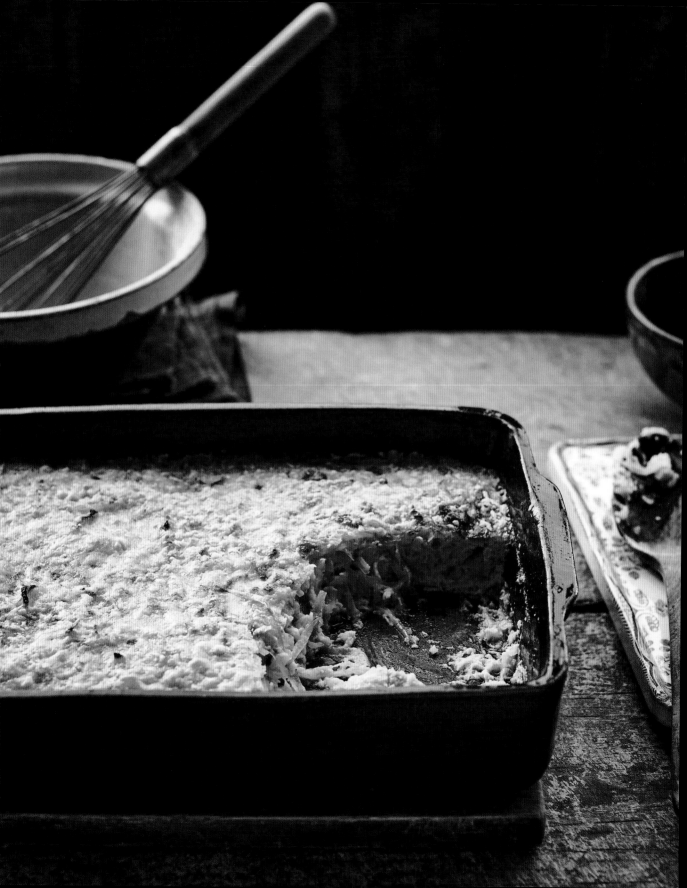

Cipolline in Agrodolce
Small Onions in Sweet and Sour Sauce

Ideally this recipe should be made with the sweet, squat, white onions, which are less strong than pickling onions, and which are in season in the autumn. If you use pickling onions, you can get rid of some of their piquancy by first peeling and then soaking them in cold water for about 1 hour.

Serves 4

750g/1lb 10oz small white onions

25g/1oz/½ tbsp unsalted butter

2 tbsp olive oil

1 tbsp tomato purée (paste)

1½ tbsp caster sugar

2 tbsp wine vinegar

Sea salt and freshly ground black pepper

Prepare the onions by plunging them into boiling water for a few minutes which makes it easier to peel them. Remove, leave until cool enough to handle and then peel them. Be careful not to remove the roots or the onions will break during cooking.

Heat the butter and oil in a large frying pan, into which the onions can fit in more or less a single layer. When the butter has melted and starts fizzing add the onions and stir them around for a minute before adding the tomato purée. Then pour in about 50ml/2fl oz/3½ tbsp of hot water. Mix very thoroughly and cook, uncovered, over a very gentle heat, for 30 minutes, adding more hot water whenever necessary during the cooking.

Turn the heat up and add the sugar. Let the onions caramelize in the sugar for a minute or two and then add the wine vinegar and season with salt and pepper. Mix well, turn the heat down and continue cooking for about 1 hour, adding more hot water whenever the onions look too dry. The onions are ready when they are a rich brown colour and can easily be pierced by the point of a knife.

These onions are delicious warm as an accompaniment to roast chicken, steak or a plain frittata. They can also be served cold as part of an antipasto.

Cipollata
Onion Soup

Serves 4

3 tbsp extra virgin olive oil

800g/1lb 12oz onions, very finely sliced

1 tsp sugar

1 x 400g/14oz can chopped tomatoes

1 litre/1¾ pints/4 cups vegetable or chicken stock

1cm/½in piece fresh red chilli (chili), deseeded and finely sliced

4 slices sourdough bread

1 garlic clove

12 basil leaves, torn in little bits

Freshly grated mature pecorino to serve

Sea salt and freshly ground black pepper

There are many onion soup recipes in Italy, some with cheeses, as in Piedmont, some with cabbage, others with farro. It was difficult to choose just one recipe for this book, but I decided on this one, which originates from Umbria. I found it in a delightful little book written by a nun; that's all I remember since, unfortunately, I lost the original book during one of my moves. It was one of the recipes I included in my second cookery book *The Good Housekeeping Italian Cookery* (1982). Pecorino is better than Parmesan cheese for this soup because of its stronger flavour.

Put the oil in a heavy-based pan and add the onions, sugar and 2 pinches of salt. Cover the pan with a lid and cook at the gentlest heat for about 1 hour, turning over the onions frequently and, if necessary, adding a little boiling water. At the end the onion should resemble a mash.

Add the tomatoes, stock and chilli and bring to the boil. Stir and cook over a low heat for another 30 minutes. Taste and check the salt and add pepper if necessary, although you might find it hot enough because of the chilli.

Before serving, toast or grill the bread slices and then rub them with the garlic clove, cut in half. Place one slice in each bowl. Ladle the soup over the bread and sprinkle with the basil. Hand the pecorino around in a bowl.

Coste
Swiss chard

Coste is not the proper name of this vegetable; it should be *bietole costa*, but this is not a botanical book and I prefer to use the colloquial word.

Swiss chard is one of the vegetables I rely on in the autumn and early winter. I use locally grown Swiss chard which I never get bored of cooking in many different ways. I usually cut off the green leaves and use them as I would spinach, while I cook the white ribs in many different ways — my favourite remains the classic method of baking them sometimes with béchamel sauce, sometimes not, but always with plenty of cheeses.

Bietole Strascinate al Pomodoro
Swiss Chard in Tomato Sauce

Serves 4

1kg/2lb 4oz Swiss chard, leaves only

3 tbsp extra virgin olive oil

2 garlic cloves, chopped

4 anchovy fillets, drained

1 tsp chilli (chili) flakes

3 ripe tomatoes, peeled and chopped

*Sea salt and freshly ground black
   pepper*

Wash the leaves thoroughly, drain and cut them into strips.

In a sauté pan heat the oil, then add the garlic, anchovy fillets and chilli and sauté for 3–4 minutes, while pressing the mixture hard into the bottom of the pan with a metal spoon to mash the anchovies.

Add the tomatoes with all their juices to the pan and continue cooking for 5 minutes. Now add the Swiss chard leaves and mix well. Cover the pan and sauté until tender, which takes longer than you think – some 15 minutes or more. Stir occasionally and add a little hot water every now and then to prevent the chard sticking to the bottom of the pan. When the chard leaves are tender if there is too much liquid in the pan, just remove the lid, and cook over a high heat until it has partly evaporated. Taste and check the seasoning. Serve hot or at room temperature.

Coste al Gratin
Swiss Chard Bake

Serves 4

1kg/2lb 4oz Swiss chard, ribs only

100g/3½oz fontina or fontal

25g/1oz/1½ tbsp unsalted butter

2 eggs

2 tbsp milk

4 tbsp freshly grated Parmesan

*Sea salt and freshly ground black
   pepper*

Heat the oven to 160°C Fan/180°C/350°F/Gas Mark 4.

Wash the ribs in plenty of water, removing all the earth which is often stuck in the ribs. Drain and cut them into 10cm/4in pieces. Bring a saucepan of water to the boil, add 1 tbsp of salt and the ribs. Cook for about 5–7 minutes until tender. Drain well and dry with kitchen paper.

Cut the fontina or fontal in thin slices. Take a Swiss chard rib and place a slice of the cheese into it. Cover with another rib, so as to make a sandwich. Repeat with the rest of the ribs. Generously butter a large, rectangular, ovenproof dish and cover the bottom with a layer of Swiss chard sandwiches. If your dish is not large enough to accommodate them all, make two layers of sandwiches.

Beat the eggs with the milk and mix in the Parmesan, salt and pepper. Spoon this mixture over the Swiss chard sandwiches, taking care that the egg mixture runs between each sandwich. Place the dish in the oven and bake for 15 minutes, until a golden crust has formed on top. Leave the dish to stand for a few minutes before serving.

Fagiolini
Green beans

Fagiolini arrived in Europe late from the New World – in the 17th century – but, once here, they became a favourite from north to south. In Italy they quickly became a popular crop and many varieties were developed, ranging in colour from ivory to purple and all through the different greens, and size, from 10–50cm/4–20in. *Fagiolini di Sant' Anna* are the longest beans, so called because they are ready to be harvested on that saint's name day of 26 July. Because of their name, they were my favourite beans when I was a child. And Maria, our cook, used to leave one whole green bean in all its length and put it on my plate, like a long, thin, coiled snake which I could then, with great delight, cut up myself.

It is impossible to say how long green beans take to cook, because it depends on how they were grown. The more natural their cultivation the longer they take to be ready. In recent years it has become fashionable to eat green beans while still crunchy, a fashion which I detest. I want my beans to be just firm but not too stiff or squeaky. When I cook them, I know that they are ready when I can detect an aroma coming from the saucepan in which they are cooking.

Green beans are usually first blanched by steaming or boiling and then either eaten at room temperature in a salad or they undergo a second cooking, either being gently fried in olive oil and butter or cooked in a tomato sauce. Fresh, young beans can also be cooked from raw in a thin tomato sauce. They take a long time to cook in this way and some care is required, since a little liquid might have to be added at various times during the cooking.

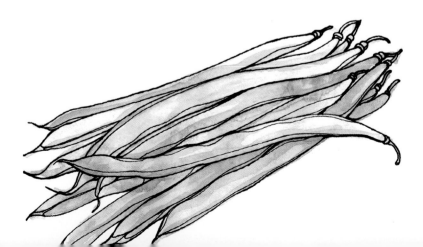

Fagiolini col Prosciutto Cotto e Grana
Green Bean, Ham and Grana Padano Salad

This is more of a main course than a side dish. Buy the ham cut in a single thick slice, because you need thick pieces in the salad.

Serves 2
400g/14oz green beans
1 thick slice of ham, about 120g/4½oz
A squeeze of lemon juice
About 25g/1oz Grana Padano, shaved

For the dressing
1 heaped tsp French mustard
4 tbsp extra virgin olive oil
1 tbsp wine vinegar
Sea salt and freshly ground black
pepper

Top and tail the green beans and wash them in plenty of water. Cook them by steaming them or boiling them in plenty of salted water until they are done to your liking. I like mine cooked just firm but not so they are stiff and squeaky. As soon as they are done, refresh them under cold water, which helps to keep the green colour. Turn them into a salad bowl and cut any long beans in half. They all should be more or less 5–7cm/2–2¾in long.

Cut the ham slice into sticks, about 2cm/¾in wide and 5–7cm/2–2¾in long, and mix into the beans.

Now prepare the dressing or *salsina*. In a small bowl, put the French mustard and slowly add the oil, while beating with a fork to emulsify the sauce – a fork is better than a spoon. Slowly add the vinegar and a little pepper while continuing to beat the whole time. Spoon this *salsina* over the beans and mix thoroughly. Squeeze a little lemon juice over the salad and mix again. Taste and adjust the salt, but remember that you still have to add the cheese, which is naturally salty.

Mix half the shaved Grana Padano into the salad, sprinkling the remainder on top just before serving. I usually leave the dressed salad to rest for half an hour before serving so that the beans and ham can absorb the *salsina*.

Fagiolini alla Fiorentina
Green Beans in Fennel–Flavoured Tomato Sauce

In Tuscany fennel grows wild in the countryside and it is used to flavour quite a few dishes, the most famous of them all being *porchetta* or spit-roasted piglet. Alas, fennel does not grow wild in the English countryside, but it grows very well in gardens. We have two large fennel bushes in our garden in Dorset and I use some of their fronds when making this dish.

A few chopped fronds have a more delicate flavour than fennel seeds, so use fronds if you can. Alternatively, you can also use the fronds of fennel bulbs, as long as they are fresh enough. I use fennel seeds in the recipe here because they are more easily available.

Serves 4

4 tbsp extra virgin olive oil
500g/1lb 2oz green beans
1 small onion, finely sliced
1 garlic clove, finely chopped
1 x 400g/14oz can chopped plum
*   tomatoes*
1 tsp sugar
150ml/5fl oz/²⁄₃ cup vegetable stock
1 tsp fennel seeds
Sea salt and freshly ground black
*   pepper*

Top and tail the green beans and wash them in plenty of water.

Take a large sauté pan, add the oil and heat it. When it is hot, add the onion, garlic and a pinch or two of salt and cook gently until the onion is just colouring. Stir frequently.

Now add the tomatoes, sugar, salt and pepper, and cook over a lively heat for about 10 minutes. Keep an eye on it and add a little hot water if the sauce is becoming too dry.

Pour in the stock, mix well and add the beans, salt and fennel seeds, or chopped fronds if using. Mix thoroughly, cover the pan and cook gently until done, which will take at least 30 minutes. Green beans take longer to cook when they cook in a little liquid as in this recipe. Halfway through the cooking add some boiling water so that the beans are always cooking in a little liquid. When cooked to your liking, taste, adjust the seasoning and serve.

Fagiolini e Patate al Pesto
Green Beans and Potatoes with Pesto

This is not a dish you will ever see in Italy, or maybe very rarely, but I have decided to include it in this book because of the popularity of pesto in Britain. While in Italy pesto is eaten only with pasta, here it is matched with many other ingredients.

In Liguria, the motherland of basil pesto, a few cubed potatoes and cut up French beans are boiled in the water together with the pasta. The drained mixture is then dressed with pesto. Here I have eliminated the pasta and written the recipe just for beans and potatoes. And it is delicious.

If you don't feel like making pesto from scratch, use a good brand of ready made pesto. I sometimes use Sacla pesto to which I add a bit of extra garlic and 1 tbsp of my best oil.

Serves 6
500g/1lb 2oz new potatoes
500g/1lb 2oz green beans
1 tbsp extra virgin olive oil
3 tbsp pine nuts
Sea salt

For the pesto
25g/1oz basil leaves
1 garlic clove
3 tbsp extra virgin olive oil
1 tbsp lemon juice

Scrub the potatoes, put them in a saucepan and cover with water. Bring the water to the boil. Add 1 tbsp of salt and cook until the potatoes are tender when pricked with the point of a knife. Drain and set aside. If you want, remove the skins as soon as the potatoes are cool enough to handle. Personally I never peel new potatoes.

While the potatoes are cooking, top and tail and wash the beans. Cut them in half and drop them in a saucepan of boiling, salted water. Cook them to your liking. I like my green beans to be just firm, not squeaky. When they are ready, drain them well and transfer them to a bowl.

Cut any large potatoes into halves or quarters and add to the beans. Toss the whole thing with the olive oil and set aside.

Dry fry the pine nuts in a non-stick frying pan. Be careful not to burn them which is quite easy. As soon as they are a golden colour, add to the beans and potatoes.

To make the pesto, finely chop the basil leaves with the garlic and then gradually add the oil while beating with a fork. Pour in the lemon juice, spoon the dressing over the potatoes and mix together very thoroughly. Taste and check the salt. Pepper is not usually added to pesto, but you can add it if you want.

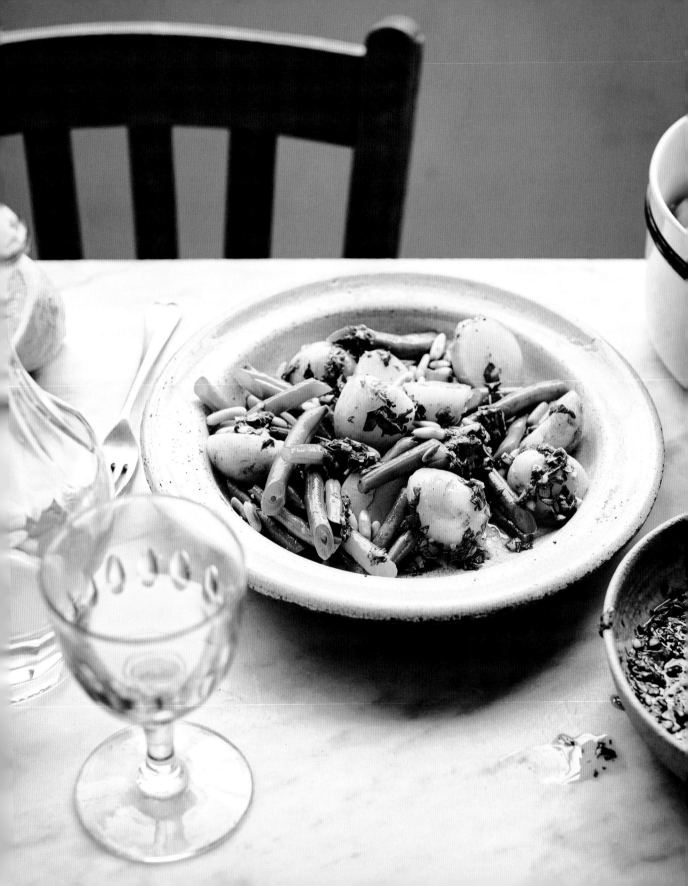

Torta di Fagiolini e Coste
Green Beans and Swiss Chard Cake

The origins of this cake are hardly Italian since the recipe was created by my friend Michelle Berriedale-Johnson in her kitchen in Belsize Park, London. Michelle based her cake on my *Sformato di Spinaci* or Spinach Mould (see page 164) and adapted it a little. Now in my kitchen in Dorset, I have slightly changed her version. No cook can ever make a dish without adding her own twist – a sort of signature.

Serves 6

400g/14oz fine green beans

1 large leek

2 x 30g/1oz cans of anchovies in oil

4 tbsp olive oil

400g/14oz Swiss chard, ribs and leaves washed and chopped into small pieces

6 large (US extra-large) eggs

50g/1¾oz/scant 1 cup fresh white breadcrumbs

5 tbsp freshly grated Parmesan

Freshly ground black pepper

Heat the oven to 160°C Fan/180°C/350°F/Gas Mark 4. Line a 25cm/10in cake tin with baking parchment.

Top and tail the beans, wash them and cut them in half. Steam the beans for 3–4 minutes until they have softened slightly but still have some crunch. Set aside.

Remove the green foliage from the leek and discard (keep it for a soup). Slice the white bulb very finely and wash thoroughly.

Chop the anchovies and put them in a frying pan with their oil, the olive oil and leek. Cook gently for 5–8 minutes, pressing down the mixture with the back of the spoon to reduce the mixture to a mush.

Meanwhile, steam the Swiss chard for 3–4 minutes. As with the beans, you want to soften it but still retain some texture.

Tip the beans and the chard into the leek mixture and sauté for 5 minutes, turning the mixture over and over. Transfer to a bowl. Beat the eggs and add to the mixture, followed by the breadcrumbs and the cheese. Mix together thoroughly and season generously with freshly ground black pepper (you should not need any salt because of the anchovies and the cheese), then spoon into the cake tin. Smooth off the top.

Place in the oven and bake for 45 minutes or until a wooden stick or a piece of dried spaghetti inserted into the middle of the cake comes out dry. Remove from the oven and leave to cool slightly. Then unmould the cake onto a plate. Serve at room temperature with the *Pomodorini Arrostiti* (see page 137) or surrounded by scrambled eggs for a perfect supper meal.

Fagioli
Beans

We owe the New World many good things including the introduction to Europe of some of our most loved vegetables, among which are beans in all their many varieties.

The first beans were cultivated in Italy at the beginning of the 16th century. The two most popular Italian varieties are borlotti from Veneto and cannellini from Tuscany. Both are usually sold dried and they must be soaked in water before cooking. But they are even more delicious fresh as they have a stronger flavour – they cook in about 30 minutes. Borlotti beans are usually used in soups, while cannellini beans are perfect in salads or a stew. There is one variety, the *fagioli dall'occhio* (black-eyed bean), which has been cultivated in Europe since Etruscan times. They are very good but no longer very popular.

Fava
Broad bean

Years ago we had an old farmhouse in Chianti, in Tuscany. We only had enough money to restore the first floor, leaving the ground floor as it was, all arches and stones and brambles, very beautiful but not very habitable unless you were a pig. We stayed there every Easter to enjoy the first warm sun of the year and the first broad beans. On Easter Sunday we always went to have lunch at the trattoria just up the road where Gino, the proprietor, was happy to squeeze us in no matter how many customers he already had. As soon as we sat down at our table, he placed three things in front of us: a flask of Chianti, a round of pecorino and a bowl of fresh broad beans. *'Eccoci e buon appetito'* and left us to the pleasure of eating those small greeny pearls popped out of their pods. And what an antipasto that was.

If you are using fresh beans in their pod you need to start with approximately four times the weight of podded beans required. This will vary, depending on how full the pod and how big the beans. Frozen beans work well, too – use the same weight for both fresh and frozen beans.

Broad beans should be boiled and peeled before you can do anything with them. I always remove the skins from cooked broad beans, because I dislike the bits of skin under my teeth. You might be less fussy and this will cut down some of the preparation time.

Insalata di Tonno e Cannellini
Cannellini Beans and Tuna Salad

Cannellini are often used in salads, and this is one of the most popular dishes. It is supposed to originate from Livorno – which is oddly translated as Leghorn in English – where some of the best canned tuna is prepared. Buy the best canned tuna you can, which is usually sold in jars. Cheap tuna can ruin everything.

If you prefer a less strong taste of spring onions, as I do, after having cut them in rings, let them soak for at least half an hour in boiling, salted water. Drain and rinse them and then proceed as in the recipe.

Serves 4

1 x 200g/7oz can cannellini beans

4 tbsp extra virgin olive oil

Juice of 1 unwaxed lemon

250g/9oz tuna preserved in olive oil

4 spring onions (scallions)

1 tsp Dijon mustard

25g/1oz/1 cup flat leaf parsley,
    chopped

Sea salt

Drain the cannellini beans, rinse them and put them in a salad bowl. Mix in 2 tbsp of the oil and a squeeze of lemon juice. Flake the tuna and add to the bowl.

Wash the spring onions, remove the roots and discard, and slice them thinly. Add to the bowl and mix well using two forks.

Put the remaining oil in a bowl, add 1 tbsp of lemon juice and the mustard and beat well with a fork. You could include a small amount of the tuna oil in the dressing if you want. Pour the dressing over the cannellini and tuna mixture and mix again. Taste and check for salt and sprinkle the parsley over before serving.

Fagioli all'Uccelletto
Cannellini Beans Sautéed in Garlic Oil

Why this recipe is called *all'uccelleto* or 'in the manner of a bird' nobody has ever been able to explain. The most likely reason is that it is the ideal accompaniment to a roasted bird, of which the Tuscans are particularly fond. When the shooting season starts at the beginning of September the peace of the Tuscan countryside is shattered by the regular blast of shotguns. The motto is 'If it flies, shoot'. And dinner is ready accompanied by a dish of cannellini, the Tuscan beans.

This classic dish can be made with or without tomatoes. Here is the simpler, older version without tomatoes, which I prefer because the flavour of the beans comes out stronger. If you prefer the tomato version, add 400g/14oz of peeled and chopped tomatoes to the garlicky oil and cook for some 15 minutes over a lively heat before adding the beans.

It is a perfect recipe for canned cannellini beans so is quick to prepare.

Serves 4

3 garlic cloves

4 tbsp extra virgin olive oil

12 sage leaves, coarsely torn

1–2 pinches chilli flakes

2 x 400g/14oz cans cannellini beans

Sea salt

Chop the garlic cloves. If the garlic is old cut the cloves in half and remove the germ before chopping – removing the germ will make the garlic sweeter. Put the garlic in a frying pan with the oil, sage and chilli and fry gently until it begins to colour.

Drain and rinse the cannellini beans and add to the frying pan. Mix well and cook over a low heat for 5 minutes, stirring very frequently. Taste and add salt, if necessary.

Pure' di Fave con Radicchio e Cipollotti
Broad Bean Purée with Radicchio and Spring Onions

This dish originates from Puglia where it is called *incapriata*, a very odd name, indeed, which I have never been able to find out what it means. But its flavour is not odd at all; it is simply delicious.

You need dried broad beans, which you can buy in the best supermarkets or in many Middle Eastern or Italian delis. In Puglia this dish is made with the local chicory, which has a more bitter flavour than the red radicchio. I grow chicory in the garden, a solid clump of curly leaves with beautiful blue flowers; it is similar to the wild chicory from Puglia. Use chicory if you can (a handful is sufficient), otherwise use radicchio as in this recipe.

80

Serves 4

200g/7oz dried broad (fava) beans
200g/7oz waxy potatoes
1 bunch spring onions (scallions)
2 heads of red radicchio
6 tbsp extra virgin olive oil
2 tsp wine vinegar
100g/3½oz green olives, stoned
  (pitted) but not dressed
2 bay leaves
Sea salt and freshly ground black
  pepper

Soak the broad beans in cold water for 1 hour and drain. Put them in an earthenware pot that you can put directly on the heat.

Peel the potatoes, cut them into chunks and add to the broad beans. Cover with water, add 1 tbsp of salt and bring to the boil. Turn the heat down to simmer. Cook for 1 hour.

Meanwhile, cut off the green top of the spring onions, keeping only the pale green leaves and the white bulbs. Wash and cut into 1cm/½in strips. Set aside. Cut the radicchio in half and then into segments. Wash and cook it in boiling, salted water for 5 minutes. Drain.

When the broad beans and the potatoes have cooked for 1 hour, drain and transfer them to the bowl of a food processor. Whizz to a coarse purée and then scoop into a serving bowl. Mix in the radicchio, spring onion, 3 tbsp of the oil, the vinegar, salt and pepper. Taste and check the seasoning.

Heat the remaining oil in a small frying pan and, when hot, throw in the olives and the bay leaves. Cook for 5 minutes, shaking the pan frequently. Discard the bay leaves and then add the olives and the juices to the serving bowl. Serve straightaway.

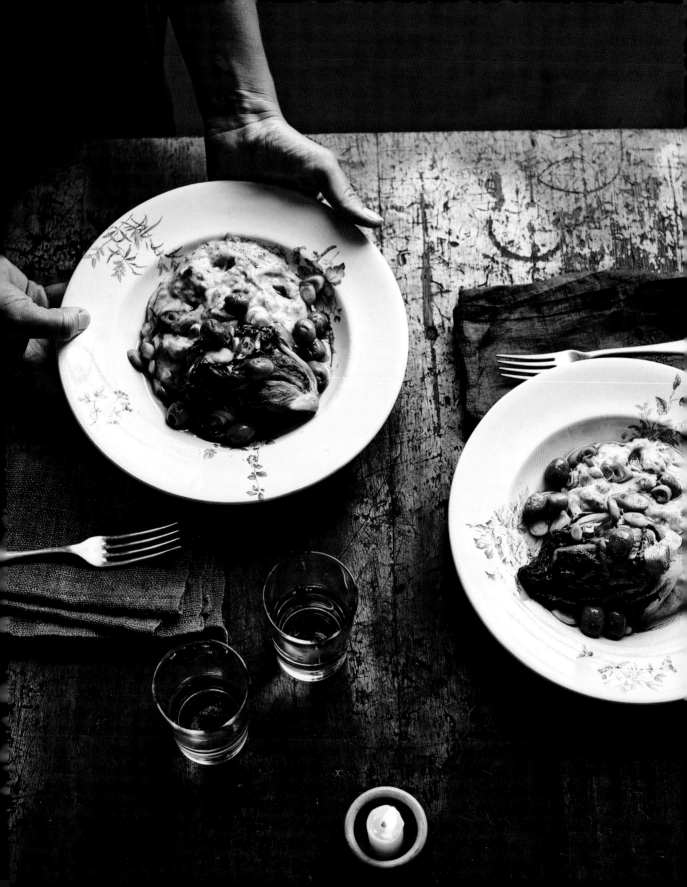

Fave con la Burrata
Broad Beans with Burrata

I first had this memorable dish at a trattoria in Puglia some 40 years ago when I was researching the first edition of my book *Gastronomy of Italy* (1987). The trattoria was a classic picture-postcard place with a terrace overlooking the blue Mediterranean Sea and the owner, in white apron, was busy telling us all his specialities, one of which was broad beans with burrata. I shamefully said to him I had never had burrata, a delicious speciality of Puglia, and he looked at me as if I was a fake cookery writer. He told me that burrata was a local speciality so fabulous that the Shah of Iran (he was still the Shah then) used to have a plane sent from Tehran to Brindisi once a week to collect enough burrata to keep him happy for the week. And that seemed quite a good recommendation. A plate was set in front of me covered by a small mountain of broad beans, on top of which sat an immaculate white ball streaked with pale green (the olive oil) and spotted with deep green (the basil). I dug my fork into it, shoved a forkful into my mouth and after just a few moments agreed that the Shah had had a very good palate.

Burrata is available in Italian delis, some supermarkets and online.

Serves 4

- *250g/9oz podded broad (fava) beans or frozen beans, thawed*
- *4 tbsp extra virgin olive oil*
- *250g/9oz burrata*
- *12 basil leaves, torn*
- *Sea salt and freshly ground black pepper*

Bring a saucepan of salted water to the boil, add the broad beans, bring the water back to the boil and cook for 2 minutes. Drain, refresh under cold water and skin them by squeezing the beans between your thumb and forefinger. This is a labour of love but it makes all the difference to the dish, especially if the beans are not all that young, as they usually are unless you can pick your own.

Put the peeled beans in a bowl, pour in 3 tbsp of the oil and season with salt and a generous grinding of black pepper. Mix well and then divide the beans among 4 individual plates.

Roughly crumble the burrata and spread equally over the broad beans. Sprinkle with the remaining oil and scatter with the basil leaves.

Fave al Guanciale
Broad Beans with Cured Pig Jowl

This is one of the most cherished recipes of Roman cuisine. The broad beans are flavoured with *guanciale*, which is a speciality of central Italy and Rome. The pig jowl is cured in the same way as pancetta, but, since the jowl is more tasty, the final result is better. You can buy *guanciale* in many Italian delis and online.

Serves 4

300g/10½oz podded broad (fava) beans or frozen beans, thawed

2 spring onions (scallions)

3 tbsp olive oil

200g/9oz guanciale

200ml/7fl oz/generous ¾ cup beef stock, homemade or made with bouillon or cube

Sea salt and freshly ground black pepper

Bring a saucepan of salted water to the boil, add the broad beans, bring the water back to the boil and cook for 2 minutes. Drain, refresh under cold water and skin them by squeezing the beans between your thumb and forefinger. This is a labour of love but it makes all the difference to the dish, especially if the beans are not all that young, as they usually are unless you can pick your own.

Trim the spring onions, remove the coarser outer leaves and the roots and cut the onions into thin slices. Wash and dry them.

Heat the oil in a saucepan, add the *guanciale* and sauté for a few minutes until crisp. Add the spring onions, cook for 1 minute and add the beans. Stir for a minute or two to coat them in the fat and then pour in about half the stock. Season with salt and pepper, cover the pan and cook, over a very low heat, for 10 minutes, turning the broad beans frequently. Add some of the remaining stock if the mixture is becoming too dry. Serve hot.

Zuppa di Fave
Broad Bean Soup

This is a lovely filling soup The ricotta added at the end brings a delicate sweetness to the soup and makes it more interesting. If you can, buy sheep's ricotta which adds a deeper flavour and a slightly tangy hint. You can find it online or in Italian, Turkish or Greek delis.

Serves 4

375–425g/13–15oz podded broad (fava) beans, or frozen beans, thawed

3 tbsp olive oil

1 onion, cut into rings

2 garlic cloves, sliced

500g/1lb 2oz ripe tomatoes, peeled and chopped

1.2 litres/2 pints/5 cups vegetable stock

1 bay leaf

2 tbsp ricotta

Sea salt and freshly ground black pepper

Bring a saucepan of salted water to the boil, add the broad beans, bring the water back to the boil and cook for 2 minutes. Drain, refresh under cold water and skin them by squeezing the beans between your thumb and forefinger. This is a labour of love but it makes all the difference to the dish, especially if the beans are not all that young, as they usually are unless you can pick your own. Set the beans aside.

Heat the oil in a saucepan, add the onion and a pinch or two of salt and sauté until just golden and soft. Add the garlic and sauté for 1 minute and then add the beans. Cook for 30 seconds, turning them over and over in the *soffritto*. Add the tomatoes and cook gently for some 8 minutes, keeping an eye on them in case they start to burn. Stir frequently.

Pour in the stock, add the bay leaf and bring to the boil. Simmer the soup for 7–8 minutes until the beans are tender. Discard the bay leaf. Add pepper to taste and adjust the seasoning. Ladle the soup into individual soup bowls and spoon ½ tbsp of ricotta into the middle of each bowl.

Pasta e Fagioli
Borlotti Bean Soup

Borlotti bean soup comes from Veneto, the region where the best borlotti grow. Every town, every village and every cook has their own special recipe. This soup is the one our cook, Maria, made for us. Maria was from the province of Udine, which is the capital of Friuli, the region next door to Veneto.

Most borlotti soups use stock made with a ham bone. Maria never used ham because, she used to say, 'Io voglio sentire il gusto dei borlotti non quello del prosciutto' (I want to enjoy the flavour of the borlotti not that of the prosciutto). So her soup was slightly lighter. The pasta she added to the soup was *maltagliati*, which means 'badly cut' and are made from the leftovers of tagliatelle, lasagne or any other homemade pasta. Since I seldom make fresh pasta nowadays, I add a few dried tagliatelle, broken into bits, or some other pasta shapes – the end of a packet, usually. The 'christening' of the extra virgin olive oil at the end is my addition. Sorry, Maria.

Fresh borlotti, if you can find them, are even better than dried. To serve 4, you will need to buy 500g/1lb 2oz of borlotti. The recipe is the same, but of course the fresh borlotti will be cooked far quicker – in about half an hour. Borlotti beans in cans or cartons are not suitable for a soup because you need the liquid in which the beans have cooked.

Serves 4

200g/7oz dried borlotti beans
1 garlic clove
The needles of 2 sprigs of rosemary
6 sage leaves
A few sprigs of flat leaf parsley
2 tbsp olive oil
100g/3½oz unsmoked pancetta cubes
2½ tbsp tomato purée (paste)
100g/3½oz tagliatelle, tagliolini or
*   ditalini*
Freshly grated Parmesan to serve
Sea salt and freshly ground black
*   pepper*

First soak the dried beans in cold water for at least 8–10 hours – overnight is ideal.

Drain and rinse the beans and put them in a heavy-based pan – an earthenware pot which can be put directly on the heat is ideal. This is because the beans must cook at the lowest heat. Pour enough water in the pot to cover the beans by about 5cm/2in. Put the pot on the heat and bring to the boil. Cover the pan and lower the heat so that the water is just simmering, using a flame diffuser under the pot, if necessary. Do not add any salt now because it tends to break the skin of the beans. When the beans are soft – which takes at least 1 hour – remove about 2 tbsp of beans using a slotted spoon and purée them in the bowl of a food processor or in a liquidizer. Set aside.

Chop together the garlic, rosemary needles, sage and parsley. Put the mixture along with the oil and pancetta in a frying pan. Cook for a minute, spoon in the tomato purée and cook for a few seconds. Add the bean purée and cook for another minute, stirring constantly. Add this mixture to the beans and their cooking liquid and season to taste. If there is not enough liquid add some water. Bring the soup to the boil and mix in the pasta. Cook until the pasta is done (which depends on the type you are using).

Taste and adjust the seasoning before you ladle the soup into individual soup bowls. Pour a few drops of your best olive oil on top of the soup and serve with the cheese.

Finocchio
Fennel

Florence fennel is the large, whitish bulb which is sometimes called by its Italian name of *finocchio*. I am not talking about the seeds or herb which have a very wide use in sweet-making, salame-flavouring or in medicaments for digestion and the like.

The large, white bulb is either round or slightly elongated. 'It greatly resembles in appearance the largest size celery, perfectly white and there is no vegetables equals it in flavour. It is eaten at dessert crude, and with and without dry salt; indeed, I preferred it to any other vegetable or to any fruit', wrote the American Consul in Livorno (Leghorn) in the late 18th century when he sent seeds to Thomas Jefferson for him to plant at his estate of Monticello in Virginia. And I totally agree, although I prefer cooked fennel to raw fennel.

Some cookery writers and chefs claim that the round bulb – also known as the female bulb – is better raw while the long bulb – the male one – is the one to eat cooked. But like many other cookery writers, I find no difference in the flavour, which is always deliciously refreshing.

Finocchi Ubriachi
Fennel Cooked in Wine, or Tipsy Fennel

Serves 4

5-6 fennel bulbs, depending on size

2 tbsp extra virgin olive oil

2 garlic cloves

100ml/3½fl oz/scant ½ cup dry white
    wine

Sea salt and freshly ground black
    pepper

This delicious but simple recipe for fennel is named *ubriachi* or 'tipsy',
after the soft fennel which is beautifully enveloped in a winey sauce.

Prepare the fennel by removing the stalks and paring away any bruised or old
parts of the outside leaves. Cut the bulbs lengthwise in quarters and wash.

Add the fennel, 100ml/3½fl oz/⅓ cup of hot water, the oil, garlic, wine, salt
and a generous grating of pepper to a saucepan. Place on the heat, cover
the pan and bring to the boil. Simmer gently for about 20 minutes until the
fennel is tender. If there is too much liquid in the pan when the fennel is
ready, lift out the fennel, put to one side and reduce the liquid over a high
heat. If the pan is short of liquid, add a little hot water during the cooking.
Remove the garlic and discard, check the seasoning and serve.

Finocchi alla Parmigiana
Baked Fennel

Serves 4

5–6 fennel bulbs, depending on size

40g/1½oz/3 tbsp unsalted butter

4 tbsp freshly grated Parmesan

2 tbsp dried breadcrumbs

Sea salt and freshly ground black
    pepper

I love fennel in every shape and form but this is probably my favourite
way of cooking it, as well as being one of the easiest.

Heat the oven to 180°C Fan/200°C/400°F/Gas Mark 6.

Trim the fennel bulbs at the base, remove the stalks and any bruised or
tough outside parts (reserve them for a soup). Cut each bulb lengthwise into
quarters and wash them. Cook the fennel in a saucepan of boiling, salted
water until just soft. It should be just tender, neither hard nor floppy. Drain
and dry the fennel.

Melt the butter in a small saucepan and as soon as it is melted, remove the
pan from the heat. Generously brush a medium-sized, ovenproof dish with
some of the melted butter and place the fennel quarters in the dish. Mix
together the cheese and the breadcrumbs, add pepper if required, sprinkle
over the fennel and pour the remaining butter over.

Place the dish in the oven and bake for 15–20 minutes until a golden crust
appears on the fennel. Remove from the oven and leave to stand for a few
minutes before serving.

Insalata di Finocchio, Funghi e Pecorino
Fennel, Mushroom and Pecorino Salad

This is a perfect, simple antipasto for the autumn when wild mushrooms are available. The best ones are ceps, but any wild mushrooms will do, as long as they are still firm. However, if you want to make the salad out of season use chestnut mushrooms, which work just as well.

Serves 4

1 fennel bulb
225g/8oz wild mushrooms
Juice of 1 unwaxed lemon
6 tbsp extra virgin olive oil
100g/3½oz pecorino
Sea salt and freshly ground black
*   pepper*

Trim the fennel bulb at the base, remove the stalks and, if necessary, pare off any brown bits or tough outer leaves. Cut the bulb vertically in half and then thinly slice it. Put in a colander and wash under cold water. Roughly dry with kitchen paper and transfer to a salad bowl.

Now prepare the mushrooms. Detach the stems from the caps and set the stems aside for another dish, such as a soup or stew. Wipe the caps clean with kitchen paper and slice them finely. Add to the fennel and drizzle with the lemon juice and half the olive oil. Season with a little salt, not too much because of the saltiness of the cheese, and a lot of freshly ground black pepper. Mix very thoroughly.

Remove the crust from the pecorino and shave the cheese into the salad. Drizzle with the rest of the oil and set the salad aside for about 30 minutes, so that the dressing is absorbed. Taste and adjust the seasoning and serve.

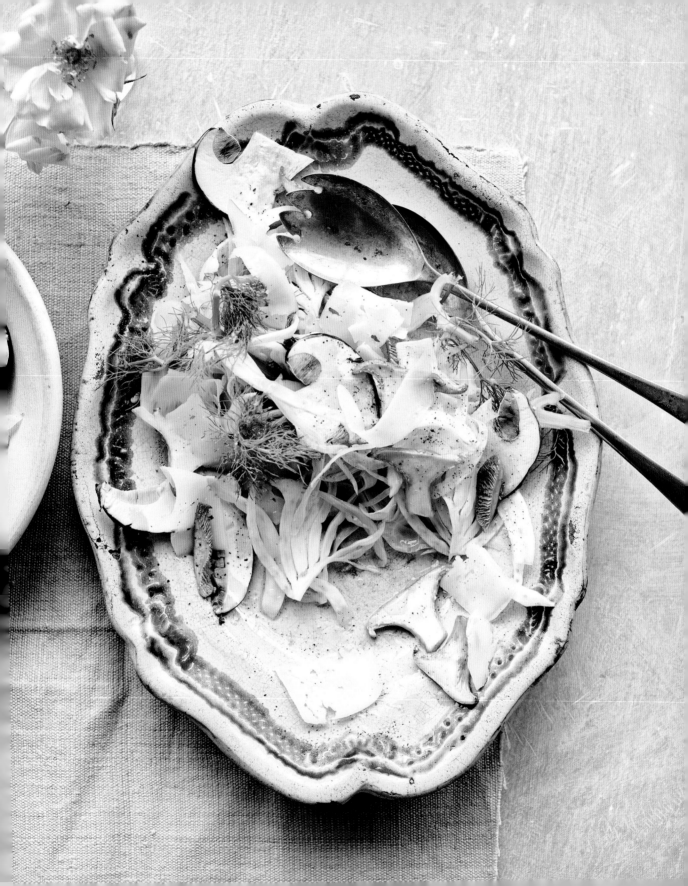

Insalata di Finocchi alla Siciliana
Fennel, Blood Orange and Black Olive Salad

This salad from Sicily is not only delicious, but is also pretty to look at, which is an added pleasure. Try to buy Italian fennel bulbs, the best on the market – or am I prejudiced?

Serves 4

2 fennel bulbs

3 blood oranges

Juice of ½ lemon

5 tbsp extra virgin olive oil

Sea salt

2 dozen black olives, stoned (pitted)

Remove the stalks and any bruised or brown parts from the fennel bulbs. Reserve the green fronds for decoration at the end, if you want. Cut the bulbs in half lengthwise and then finely slice across. Put the slices in a basin of cold water and wash. Drain thoroughly, dry with kitchen paper and transfer to a serving bowl.

Peel the oranges to the quick, which means that you must remove the skin and the white pith. Cut the oranges on a plate, to collect the juices to pour over the fennel. Cut any large orange slices in half and add to the bowl.

Pour the lemon juice onto the fennel salad. Toss, add the oil and salt to taste and toss again. Pepper is not added to this salad as it would clash with the sweetness of the oranges. Leave for 30 minutes before scattering the olives (and green fronds, if desired) on top and serve.

Finocchi al Latte
Fennel Braised in Milk

Serves 2

2 fennel bulbs, trimmed of foliage and cut in half

Sea salt

25g/1oz/1½ tbsp unsalted butter

5 tbsp milk

3 tablespoons freshly grated Parmesan

Fennel is widely available and the quality is usually very good. It goes very well with roast or grilled meats or with frittata.

Slice the fennel horizontally. Wash and dry with kitchen paper.

Bring a large saucepan of salted water to the boil and cook the fennel for 5–7 minutes until tender. Drain.

Heat the grill/broiler.

Melt the butter in a frying pan, add the fennel and cook very gently for 1 minute on each side, until soft but not coloured. Add the milk, cook gently for 5 minutes, stirring frequently, and then transfer to an ovenproof dish. Sprinkle with Parmesan and place under the hot grill for 2 minutes for the cheese to brown.

Right: Insalata di Finocchi alla Siciliana

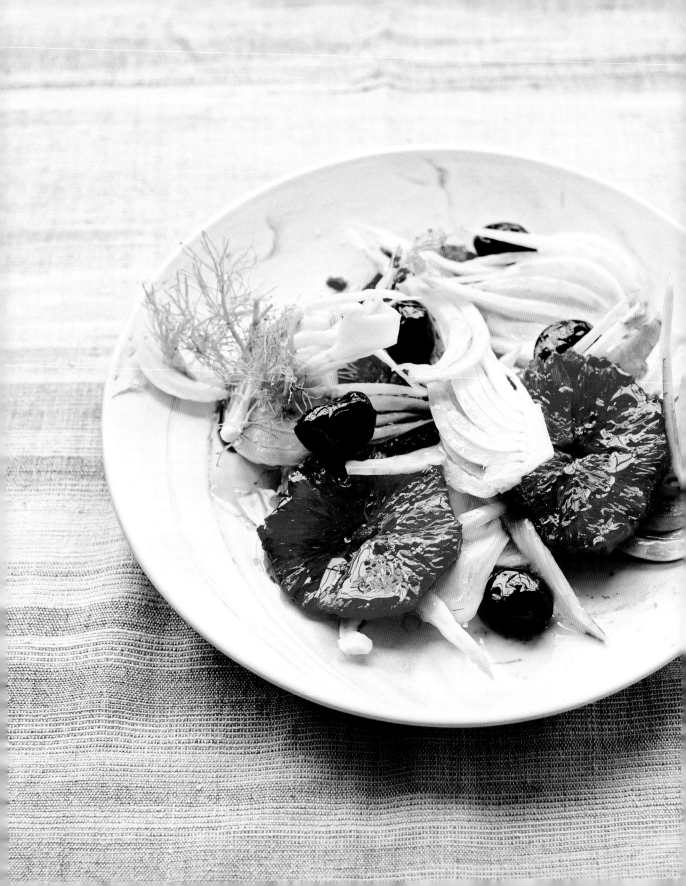

Funghi
Mushrooms

Years ago I wrote the recipes for a book on mushrooms – the book was written by a mycologist, who described what sort of mushroom you could enjoy without any fear of even the lightest tummy ache. Throughout the autumn of that year I was out every day in the open spaces of south-west London – Richmond Park, Wimbledon Common, Putney Heath, East Sheen Common and any bits of green grass in between – dressed in Wellington boots and armed with a small knife and a big basket, my eyes glued to the ground. Back home, the selection took place (edible one side and non edible the other). And then began the fun of cooking our chosen mushrooms. The fun was over pretty soon, because I discovered that really good mushrooms are very few indeed – the rest are not worth bothering with.

The best mushrooms were certainly the porcini – *Boletus edulis*, fat and juicy with that earthy truffle flavour – but I rarely found enough of them. I might also have found some chanterelles or some other kinds of boletus, a few young parasols and some field or horse mushrooms.

I don't go mushroom foraging any longer – it is not a sport for nonagenarians – but I still enjoy cooking and eating them. In the absence of wild ones, I use cultivated – chestnut mushrooms are the best. I usually add a few dried porcini to my recipes which I soak beforehand, using also the liquid in which they have soaked.

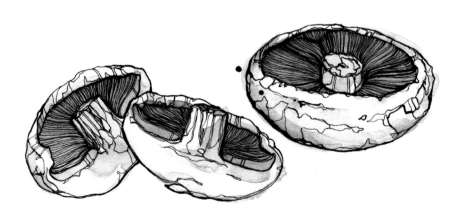

Funghi Trifolati
Sautéed Mushrooms

If you make this recipe in autumn you can use wild mushrooms. Here, I have used cultivated mushrooms and dried porcini so that it can be made all the year round – the dried porcini give the sauce the necessary mushroomy taste.

Sautéed mushrooms are a good accompaniment to roast chicken or to the *Sformato di Spinaci* (Spinach mould) recipe (see page 164). They also make an excellent pasta sauce – dress the drained pasta with 2 tbsp of oil and then mix in the mushrooms. I love sautéed mushrooms on polenta, too.

Serves 4–6

15g/½oz dried porcini
4 tbsp extra virgin olive oil
30g/1oz/2 tbsp unsalted butter
2 garlic cloves, chopped
2 tbsp chopped marjoram leaves
2 tbsp chopped flat leaf parsley
500g/1lb 2oz mixed cultivated
  mushrooms, sliced
Sea salt
1 tbsp tomato purée (paste)
200ml/7fl oz/generous ¾ cup dry white
  wine
Freshly ground black pepper

Put the dried porcini in a bowl and cover with boiling water. Set aside for 20 minutes or so to soften. When the time comes, lift them out gently from the liquid and chop them coarsely. Reserve the liquid for later.

Heat the oil and the butter in a large sauté pan and, when the butter begins to become gold, add the garlic and the herbs and fry for 2 minutes. Do not let the garlic burn. Add the dried porcini and cook for about 2–3 minutes.

Now add the sliced mushrooms, a large handful at a time, allowing them to wilt between each addition, and a small pinch of salt. Cook, stirring, for about 2 minutes and then mix in the tomato purée and stir again for 1 minute. Pour in the wine and, very gently, the porcini liquid – add this very slowly so that if there is any grit at the bottom of the bowl, you leave it behind. Mix well, season with pepper and bring to the boil. Cover the pan and turn the heat down. Cook for 30 minutes and then taste to see if the mushrooms are done to your liking. Serve hot or warm as an antipasto.

Zuppa di Funghi e Orzo
Wild Mushroom and Pearl Barley Soup

I have always made this soup with wild mushrooms, either ones that I have picked myself or ones given to me by kind friends. Last week I made it with a perfect puffball of about 500g/1lb 2oz. I sliced one half, breadcoated and fried it and, with the other half, made this delicious soup. If you are not a forager, wild mushrooms are easily available to buy during the autumn.

You can also make the soup with cultivated brown mushrooms with the help of some 25g/1oz of dried porcini for the necessary stronger flavour.

Serves 4

1 onion, finely chopped

1 tbsp olive oil

250–300g/9–10½oz wild mushrooms

½ tbsp tomato purée (paste)

1.4 litres/2½ pints/6 cups vegetable or chicken stock

120g/4½oz pearl barley

25g/1oz/1 cup marjoram leaves, chopped

Sea salt and freshly ground black pepper

Add the onion to a stockpot with the oil and a pinch or two of salt. Cover the pot and cook over a very low heat – the onion should just become soft, not coloured at all. Add a little hot water during the cooking, which will take about 20 minutes.

Wipe the mushrooms clean with kitchen paper and chop them into 1cm/½in cubes. Add to the onion and continue cooking slowly for a further 10 minutes, stirring very frequently.

Spoon the tomato purée into the pot and cook over a higher heat for 1 minute, stirring constantly and then pour in the stock. Cover the pot and bring to the boil.

Rinse the pearl barley under cold water and add to the pot. Mix well and cook for about 20 minutes until done. Add salt and pepper to taste and ladle the soup into individual soup bowls. Sprinkle with a few marjoram leaves.

Lattuga
Lettuce

The most common varieties grown in Italy today are: *romana* (cos), *lattuga a cappuccio* (round) and *ricciolina* (salad bowl or curly lettuce). This last variety is also known as *la lollo*, short for Lollobrigida – after the actress Gina Lollobrigida – because of the attractive curves of its leaves. *Romana*, which is the most popular, is the crispest of all traditional lettuces and the best for salads. Nowadays crisp varieties of cabbage shape are also cultivated.

Lettuce is also used in cooking. Soup is one way of using lettuce, the oldest surviving recipe going back to the 15th century and Bartolomeo Sacchi, aka Platina, who suggests cooking it with eggs, and *agresto* or verjuice. This recipe has an interesting similarity to a Greek recipe in which cos lettuce is added to stewing lamb together with beaten eggs and lemon juice.

The 18th-century Neapolitan Vincenzo Corrado preferred his lettuces blanched and dressed with a pounded mixture of tarragon, anchovies and capers diluted in oil and vinegar. He lists six recipes for stuffed lettuce, of which my favourite is the one in prosciutto sauce. The lettuce is stuffed with a 'salpicon of sweetbreads, mushrooms, truffles, onions and herbs, bound with eggs and sautéed in veal fat and chopped prosciutto. Stuffed, they are cooked in a *coli* of prosciutto.' Another recipe, *lattughe alla certosina*, suggests a stuffing made with fish, anchovies, herbs and spices, mixed with a purée of peas.

Lattughe ripiene is a traditional dish still made in Liguria. The inner leaves of a round lettuce are stuffed with a mixture of brains, sweetbreads, mushroom, garlic, parsley and breadcrumbs. The little bunches are tied at the top with string and braised in meat stock, with which they are served. A simpler stuffing can also be made with chopped herbs, eggs and grated pecorino and Parmesan cheeses.

One recipe from Rome combines lettuce with broad beans: the dried beans, previously soaked and boiled, are sautéed in olive oil with the lettuce and then tomatoes are added.

Insalata
Green Salad

Insalata in Italy means green salad made with lettuce, chicory, lamb's lettuce, little gems, cos, radicchio, endive and all sorts of leaves simply dressed with olive oil, wine vinegar or lemon juice and salt – pepper is very often not added, nor is garlic. Rocket is not essential, but it is often part of the selection. I don't like Iceberg lettuce.

Here is how I dress my *insalata* to which I add a small clove of garlic, or half a clove, and a bunch of herbs from the garden, whatever is there. If you don't grow any herbs at home, buy a bag of two or three different fresh herbs. I like to make the dressing some half an hour before I want to eat the salad so that the flavour of the garlic is well established.

Serves 6

A selection of green leaves, such as
    lettuce, curly endive (frisée), chicory,
    romaine, lamb's lettuce, plus a few
    leaves of red radicchio
2 tbsp red wine vinegar, or more
    according to personal taste
2 tsp fine sea salt
Freshly ground black pepper
Sorrel, borage, basil, mint (only
    2 leaves), marjoram, chives,
    dandelion, all finely chopped
1 small garlic clove or ½ clove, bruised
7 tbsp extra virgin olive oil

Wash and dry the salad and tear the leaves into smallish pieces. Only lamb's lettuce must be left whole. Salad torn into small pieces absorbs more dressing than when left in big leaves.

Put the vinegar, salt, pepper and all the chopped herbs in a salad bowl. Add the bruised garlic. Use a fork to mix well. Now gradually add the oil while you continue beating with the fork. When all the oil has been added, remove the garlic.

Add half the salad to the bowl, toss well and then add the remaining half. Toss very thoroughly. The secret of a good salad is in the tossing. Go deep with your fork and spoon to lift up and turn each piece. There is an Italian saying which goes: 'You need four people to dress a salad: a generous person to pour the oil, a wise person to add the vinegar, a mean person to season with salt and a mad person to toss it'. Another saying is that 'Salad should be tossed as many times as the years of Christ', i.e. 33 times.

That's all.

Insalata di Valerianella, Rucola e Pinoli
Lamb's Lettuce, Rocket and Pine Nut Salad

This salad brings together two type of salad from the two ends of the Italian peninsula. *Rucola* or rocket is the most characteristic green leaf of Puglia, the heel of the boot, while the *valerianella* or lamb's lettuce is very popular in northern Lombardy, where it is now widely cultivated. Lamb's lettuce consists of a cluster of bright, rather succulent leaves which are ready for picking from April onwards. It is also called *insalata pasqualina*, or Easter salad, and is the traditional salad to be served after the Paschal roast kid or lamb.

Like most children, I was not passionate about salads in general, while our mother was very much so. So green salad of most shapes and forms appeared quite often on our table. The only salad which I could eat with pleasure was the little *valerianella*, which we sometimes had with the first bright red radishes of the season. The salad was dressed with a delicate olive oil and just a little lemon juice and a pinch or two of salt – no pepper, vinegar or fruity olive oil, which would have interfered with the delicate flavour of the lamb's lettuce.

However, having just said what I have, it seems outrageous that I should now give you a recipe in which the delicate lamb's lettuce is dressed with such a spicy sauce. I apologise to the purists – of which usually I am one – but this recipe does work, I promise you.

Serves 6
400g/14oz lamb's lettuce
400g/14oz rocket (arugula)
50g/1¾oz pine nuts
8 anchovy fillets, drained
2 garlic cloves, peeled
6 tbsp extra virgin olive oil
1–2 pinches chilli (chili) flakes
Sea salt

Wash, drain and dry the two kinds of salads and set aside.

Dry fry the pine nuts in a heavy iron pan. Be careful and keep a watch on them, because it takes 2 seconds for them to burn and be ruined. The nuts should just become slightly gold. Put them in the bowl of a food processor.

Tear the anchovy fillets into bits and add to the bowl, together with the garlic, 1 tbsp of the oil and the chilli. Blitz for a few seconds; then push down all the bits into the bottom of the bowl and blitz again for a few seconds. Place the contents into a second bowl and slowly add the remaining oil while beating with a fork. Season with salt, but remember that the anchovy fillets are quite salty.

Put about 2 handfuls of the salad leaves into a large salad bowl, add 2–3 tbsp of the dressing and mix well; spoon the rest of the dressing over and mix again. Taste, adjust the salt and serve.

Lenticchie
Lentils

One of the happiest memories of my travels through Italy is the sight of the plain of Castelluccio in Umbria. We turned the corner, so to speak, and in front of us lay a carpet of a pale blue colour covering the vast plain enclosed all around by formidable peaks of gnarled rocks: the Castelluccio plain, the land of the best lentils in the world – or maybe one of the two best lentils in the world, the other being the French Puy. Castelluccio lentils are small and dark and cook very quickly. However, the more common continental lentils should not be despised.

Lentils are the oldest of all Mediterranean pulses, their origins probably going back more than 7000 years. Lentils were very popular in Roman times, so much so that, as the chickpea gave its name to the family of the orator Cicero, lentils gave their name to the powerful Lentuli family. Down the centuries, lentils have been cooked in many ways, especially as soups, often combined with rice, or just simply braised in the usual onion *soffritto*. Writing at the end of the 19th century, the great cookery writer Artusi has only two recipes for lentils, one a soup and the other a purée of lentils sautéed in the usual *soffritto*. Lentils are a delectable food with which to make soups, to serve as a *contorno* or accompaniment to a rich pork dish or to use in a salad, as it is now often done.

Buy fresh-looking dried lentils that look smooth without wrinkles and any sprouting bits. The best lentils should be eaten within 8–10 months of harvest. They are very easy to cook since they do not need any pre-soaking, unlike other pulses; just put them in a sieve and rinse them under cold water while checking for grit and stones. Actually, nowadays lentils are pretty clean when you buy them.

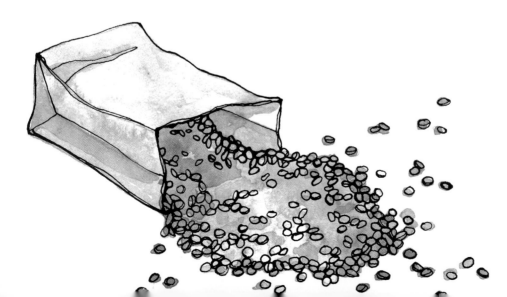

Zuppa di Lenticchie
Lentil Soup

There are two main Italian recipes for lentil soup, one from Veneto and the other from Campania. I have tried them both but I usually cook the one from Veneto, as below. The one from Campania needs the sort of tomatoes which are hard to find out of Italy.

Serves 6

500g/1lb 2oz continental lentils

50g/1¾oz anchovy fillets, drained

2 garlic cloves

6 sage leaves

15g/½oz/½ cup flat leaf parsley, main stalk removed

1 shallot

1 small celery stalk, with its leaves

100ml/3½fl oz/scant ½ cup olive oil

100g/3½oz passata (strained tomatoes)

Sea salt and freshly ground black pepper

Rinse the lentils under cold water and put them in a pot. Cover with cold water by about 4cm/1½in and bring the water to the boil. Cook for about 20 minutes until the lentils are tender. It will depend on their variety and their freshness – the longer the lentils have been stored, the longer they take to cook. Taste and see for yourself. Strain and reserve the cooking liquid.

While the lentils are cooking, put the anchovy fillets, garlic, sage, parsley, shallot and celery into the bowl of a food processor and blitz for a few seconds until everything is finely chopped. Stop the machine every so often and scrape down the sides of the bowl.

Heat the oil in a pan – I use an earthenware pot which can be put straight on the heat, because earthenware is the best material to cook pulses in. Add the anchovy mixture and sauté for 4–5 minutes, stirring frequently. Mix in the passata and sauté for a further 2 minutes and then add the lentils. Cook for 3 minutes, while stirring them around.

Measure the lentil cooking liquid and add 1.4 litres/2½ pints/6 cups to the lentils in the pot. Mix well and bring to a gentle simmer. If you don't have the full amount of cooking liquid, add boiling water to make up the amount. Taste, season with pepper, adjust the salt and serve.

Lenticchie in Umido coi Pomodori Secchi
Stewed Lentils with Sundried Tomatoes

Lentils are so often my saviour for an impromptu dinner. I always keep some canned lentils to hand; sometimes they are Puy, sometimes Castelluccio (from Italy and just as good as Puy but they are more difficult to find), and sometimes just common or garden green lentils, which take a little longer to cook but are excellent cooked as in this recipe.

Tomatoes are frequently cooked with lentils. In this recipe sundried tomatoes are used to give a stronger flavour.

This dish is a very good accompaniment to roast pork or gammon. To make a vegetarian version, eliminate the pancetta and increase the amount of oil to 5 tbsp.

Serves 4

350g/12oz continental lentils

3 tbsp olive oil

75g/2¹/₂oz unsmoked pancetta cubes

2 banana shallots, very thinly sliced

12 sage leaves, torn in pieces

150g/5¹/₂oz sundried tomatoes, ready to use

1 tbsp Marigold Swiss vegetable bouillon powder

Sea salt and freshly ground black pepper

Put the lentils in a sieve and rinse under running water. Set aside while you prepare the *soffritto*.

Heat the oil, add the pancetta and sauté for 2–3 minutes until the pancetta is golden and crisp. Add the shallots and sage and sauté for 5–7 minutes, stirring often. Add the sundried tomatoes and continue to cook for a further 2–3 minutes.

Add the lentils, and let them cook in the *soffritto* for 2–3 minutes, while you stir them around. Pour in 1 litre/1¾ pints/4 cups of hot water and season with the bouillon powder and some salt. Cook until the lentils are tender – this will take about 20 minutes for the Castelluccio and Puy varieties and a little longer for the common or garden green lentils. When they are done, season with pepper and check the salt. Serve hot.

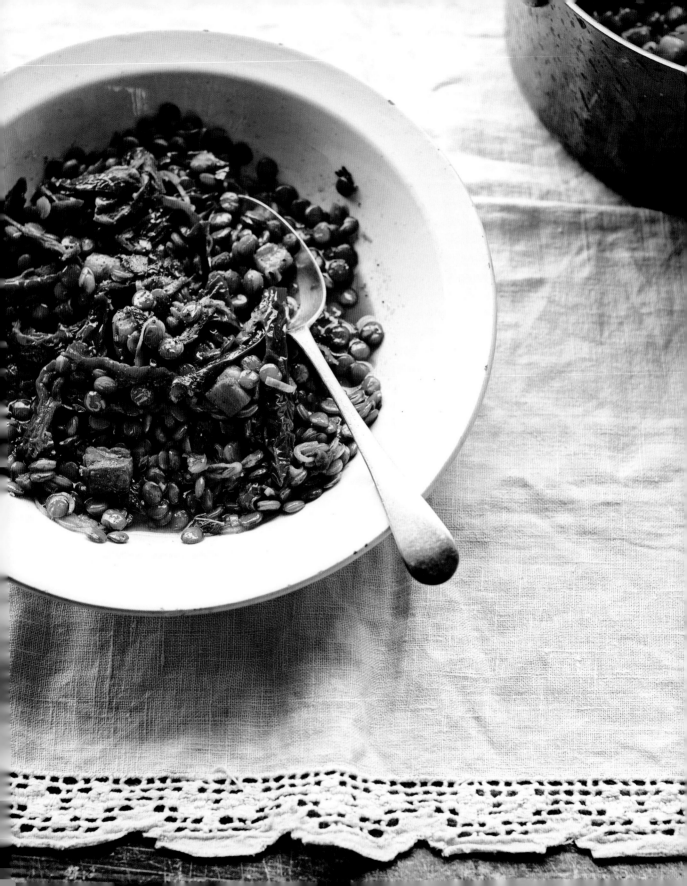

Lenticchie con la Ratatouille
Lentils in Ratatouille

Lentils are without doubt one of the best ingredients to have in the larder. They don't need presoaking, they are very versatile and they can be ready to eat in 30 minutes.

This recipe came about because my vegan granddaughter and her equally vegan American boyfriend came for supper. Feeding vegans always worries me, but as I had an ample amount of leftover ratatouille, I thought my problem was solved. I just had to cook some lentils and mix the lot together – it was easy enough and, as I discovered, very successful.

Serves 4–6

1 red onion, finely sliced

4 tbsp extra virgin olive oil

1 long pepper

1 red chilli (chili) pepper

1 aubergine (eggplant)

1 courgette (zucchini)

*1 x 400g/14oz can chopped plum
    tomatoes*

1 tbsp balsamic vinegar

For the lentils

200g/7oz continental lentils

½ onion

2 bay leaves

*Sea salt and freshly ground black
    pepper*

First prepare the ratatouille. Put the onion, oil and a pinch or two of salt in a large sauté pan and cook gently for 10 minutes.

Meanwhile, wash the pepper, cut it in half, remove the core and seeds and cut into short strips. Add the pepper to the onion. Do the same with the chilli, but cut it into very small strips. Wash the aubergine and the courgette and cut them into small cubes. Mix them a few at a time into the sauté pan. Cook for 5–6 minutes and then add the tomatoes. Season with salt and cook, uncovered, for 30 minutes. Keep a watch on the pan and add a little hot water whenever necessary. Add the balsamic vinegar and continue cooking for 30 minutes or so, until all the vegetables are soft.

While the vegetables are cooking, rinse the lentils under cold water, drain and put them in a pot. Cover them with water by some 3cm/1¼in, add the onion and bay leaves and put the pot on the heat. Bring to the boil, add salt and cook until the lentils are tender, which will vary according to the variety. Check after 20 minutes. When they are cooked, discard the onion and bay leaves.

When the ratatouille is cooked, scoop the lentils out of their liquid with a slotted spoon and add to the ratatouille a spoonful at a time. Mix well after each addition and when all the lentils have been added, cook the mixture over a low heat for 5 minutes or so to allow all the flavours to blend together.

Melanzana
Aubergine

This very versatile vegetable is of the same family as the potato and the tomato, but, unlike the latter, which reached Europe only in the 16th century, the aubergine arrived in Europe via Spain, brought there by the Arabs at the end of the first millennium. It was looked upon with suspicion due to the fact that it was a vegetable from the solanum family, which includes the poisonous nightshade. Slowly it began to be used all over Italy, albeit with suspicion. The great cookery writer Artusi wrote in 1910 in the third edition of his book *La Scienza in Cucina e l'Arte di Mangiar Bene* that aubergines and fennel were only recently available in the Florence food market; before then they had been considered as food 'suitable for the Jews'.

The aubergine travelled northwards to France and Britain and by the 17th century they were a common vegetable, probably more so in Britain than in the years following the Second World War. I remember in 1950 when I first came to London having to go all the way to Soho to buy them. But I think those years were the worst years ever in Britain as far as food goes.

Aubergines come in different shapes and colour, from small, round balls, usually of a lovely ivory-purple colour, to the oblong purple one which is the most common variety on sale in Britain. In the past aubergines were salted before cooking to get rid of some of their bitterness but nowadays this step is not necessary. However, if you are going to fry them, I recommend you salt them first; this process does rid them of some of their liquid, thus making them more brittle when fried.

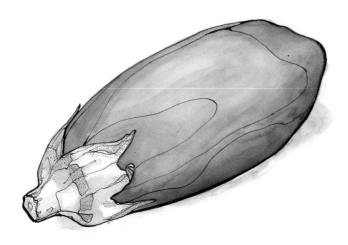

Melanzane ai Cento Sapori
Aubergines with a Hundred Flavours

This dish is the Calabrian answer to the more famous *caponata* dish from Sicily and contains, as its Sicilian counterpart often does, a little bitter chocolate.

Why it is called 'Aubergines with a Hundred Flavours' I don't know, since there are only 10 flavours, which considering the modern fashion of multiple flavourings, does not seem at all excessive. What I do know is that it is a delicious dish of aubergines bathed in flavours cleverly blended together.

Serves 4

50g/1¾oz sultanas (golden raisins)

700g/1lb 9oz aubergines (eggplant)

2 celery stalks

6 tbsp olive oil

1 onion, finely chopped

2 garlic cloves. finely chopped

2 tbsp brown sugar

3–4 tbsp wine vinegar, depending on
    strength

25g/1oz walnut kernels, chopped

25g/1oz pine nuts

25g/1oz dark chocolate

Sea salt and freshly ground black
    pepper

Put the sultanas in a bowl, cover with boiling water and leave them to plump up for some 15–20 minutes. Drain and dry them.

Remove the ends of the aubergines, wash and cut them into small cubes of about 2cm/¾in. (You can keep these smaller ends for a ratatouille or a frittata.) Remove the outside strings from the celery stalks and cut the stalks into pieces more or less the same size as the aubergine.

Take a large sauté pan and add the oil. When it is hot add the onion and garlic and cook for 5 minutes. Add the aubergines and celery and cook for a further 10 minutes, over a lively heat and stirring very frequently. Be careful that the vegetables do not catch on the bottom of the pan.

Add the sugar and let the vegetables caramelize a little before you pour in the vinegar. Cook for 5 minutes, stirring frequently, and then add the walnuts, pine nuts, sultanas and salt and pepper to taste. Mix well and continue cooking over a lively heat for 5 minutes or so, stirring frequently. The aubergines will eventually take on a golden hue.

Flake the chocolate directly over the pan. I find it is easier to use a small knife rather than a grater. Stir again and turn the heat down. Cook gently for about 45 minutes – the aubergines will be soft and the celery should still have a gentle bite. During the cooking, keep a watch on the pan and add a little hot water whenever necessary. The vegetables should always cook in a little liquid and not dry out. Taste and check the salt and pepper before serving.

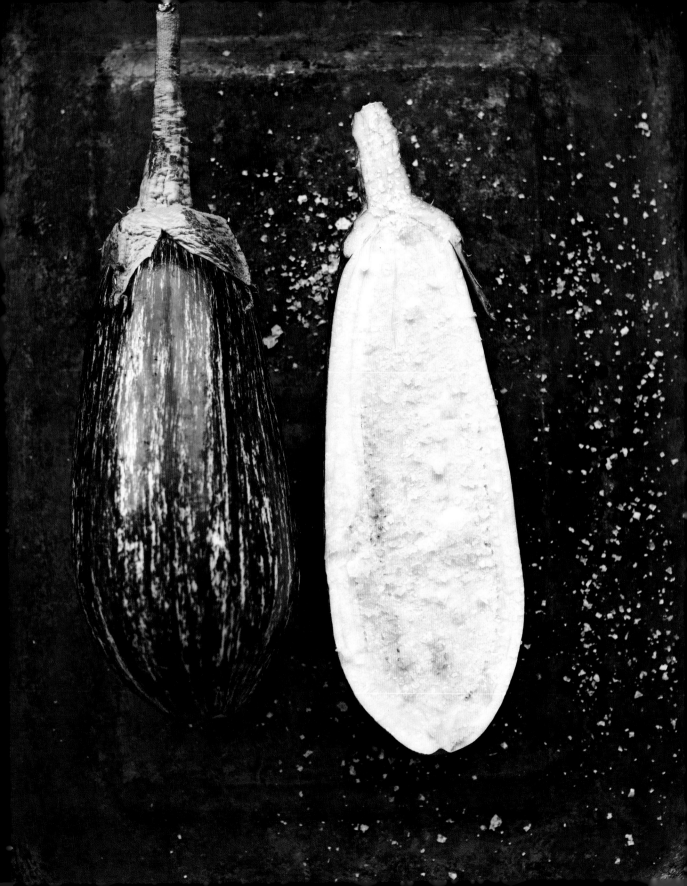

Parmigiana di Melanzane
Aubergine Parmigiana

This is one of the best Neapolitan dishes – and there are many. This recipe has been published in several of my books but it is such a classic that I feel I have to include it in this book on Italian vegetables.

Some cooks nowadays suggest roasting the aubergine slices instead of frying, probably because frying is considered to be an unhealthy method of cooking. Well, I prefer to eat *Parmigiana di Melanzane* less often, but when I do, I like it to be the original Parmigiana made with fried aubergines, as in this recipe.

Serves 4–5

1 x 400g/14oz carton passata
  (strained tomatoes)
2 garlic cloves, bruised
5 tbsp olive oil
Sea salt and freshly ground black
  pepper
1kg/2lb 4oz aubergines (eggplant)
Vegetable oil for frying
300g/10½oz Italian buffalo
  mozzarella, sliced
4 eggs, hard-boiled, shelled and sliced
12 basil leaves
5 tbsp freshly grated Parmesan
Dried breadcrumbs

First make the tomato sauce. Put the passata, garlic and 3 tbsp of the olive oil in a pan and cook over a lively heat until the oil has separated from the tomatoes. This should take about 10–15 minutes. Stir frequently and, at the end, season with salt and pepper and remove the garlic.

Meanwhile, remove the ends of the aubergines, wash them and cut them lengthwise into slices about 4–5cm/1½–2in thick. (You can keep these smaller ends for a ratatouille or a frittata.)

Pour enough vegetable oil into a large frying pan to come about 5cm/2in up the side of the pan. When very hot – it should sizzle lively when you dip a corner of the aubergine into it – add as many slices of aubergine as will fit in a single layer. Fry until a golden colour and then turn the slices over and fry the underside. Lift out the slices and place them on kitchen paper to drain.

Heat the oven to 160°C Fan/180°C/350°F/Gas Mark 4.

Brush a large lasagne dish with oil. Cover the bottom with a layer of aubergine slices, then a layer of mozzarella and sliced eggs and cover with a few blobs of tomato sauce and a sprinkling of basil leaves and grated cheese. Repeat this layering, finishing with a layer of aubergine. Mix the remaining Parmesan with the dried breadcrumbs and sprinkle the mixture over the top. Pour the remaining oil over and bake for about 30 minutes, until the top is crusty and bubbly. Allow to rest for at least 1 hour before serving. It is delicious served at room temperature, but you can warm it up before serving if you prefer.

Melanzane a Cotoletta
Fried Breaded Aubergines

A *cotoletta* is the method of frying food coated with egg and breadcrumbs. The term actually refers to a piece of meat – usually veal – which is cooked in this way. The fat used in my home in Milan – and actually in any Milanese kitchen – was butter because it is more easily absorbed by the food it is being fried with and thus it conveys its sweet flavour to the food – oil tends to form an outside film. Nowadays, for health reasons, oil is used along with butter. Oil has also the advantage of withstanding higher temperatures than butter, which is better for frying.

I love anything cooked *a cotoletta*. It is an indescribable delight to sink your teeth into the golden, crispy crust and open up a burst of different flavours, whether it be meat, fish or vegetables. Aubergine slices are perfect for the job, as are pieces of cauliflower or fennel – these need to be boiled first.

Serves 4

2 large aubergines (eggplant)
Plain flour for coating
2 eggs
75g/2¾oz dried white breadcrumbs for coating
5 tbsp freshly grated Parmesan
Sea salt and freshly ground black pepper
50g/1¾oz/4 tbsp unsalted butter
4 tbsp olive oil or vegetable oil
Lemon segments for serving

Remove the ends of the aubergines, wash and dry them and cut the aubergines lengthwise into 1cm/½in slices. (You can keep these smaller ends for a ratatouille or a frittata.)

Put the flour on a plate, break the eggs into another and the breadcrumbs and Parmesan into a third. Slightly beat the eggs together, adding a little salt and pepper.

Heat the butter and the oil in a large frying pan. Coat a slice of aubergine first in flour, then in the egg and lastly in the breadcrumb mixture. Pat the crumbs into the slice with your hands and then put it in the hot fat. Repeat with the rest of the slices and fry as many slices as will fit in in a single layer. When the underside is golden, turn over the slices and fry the other side. Remove the slices and place them on kitchen paper. Keep warm while you fry the rest and then serve them straightaway with the lemon segments.

Melanzane Ripiene alla Siciliana
Aubergines Stuffed with Bread and Tomatoes

Aubergines are perfect for stuffing, because their flavour blends so well with other flavours. This classic dish of stuffed aubergines is based on the wonderful aubergines you can buy in the Vucceria and the Ballaro', the two great food markets of Palermo in Sicily. The aubergines available here are a far cry from those sold in the Sicilian markets, but cooked in this way, they make a very good dish of utter simplicity and succulent flavour.

Serves 4

4 aubergines (eggplant)

Sea salt

Vegetable oil for frying

2 shallots, finely chopped

4 tbsp extra virgin olive oil

225g/8oz canned plum tomatoes

*1 slice white sourdough bread – about
    40g/1½oz*

1–2 garlic cloves, chopped

1 tbsp chopped flat leaf parsley

Small pinch chilli (chili) flakes

1 tbsp dried breadcrumbs

Remove the ends of the aubergines and cut them in half lengthwise. (You can keep these on for the look of the dish or use the smaller bits for a ratatouille or a frittata.) Sprinkle the cut sides with salt and leave them to drain, cut side down, on a wooden board for about 1 hour. When the time is up, dry them thoroughly with kitchen paper.

Pour enough vegetable oil into a frying pan to come about 2cm/¾in up the side of the pan. Heat the oil and when hot slide in the aubergine halves, skin side down. Fry for 5 minutes and then turn the halves over and fry for about 2–3 minutes until the flesh begins to become golden. Lift the halves out with a fish slice and place them on kitchen paper, cut side down.

Heat the oven to 180°C Fan/200°C/400°F/Gas Mark 6.

Now prepare the stuffing. Gently sauté the shallot with a pinch of salt in 1½ tbsp of the olive oil for about 5 minutes. While the shallot is frying, scoop out the flesh from the aubergine halves, leaving about 1.5cm/⅝in of flesh all the way round. Chop the flesh, add to the pan and sauté for 5 minutes, mixing frequently. Lift the tomatoes out of their juice, roughly chop them and add to the pan. Continue cooking for about 10 minutes, stirring frequently.

Meanwhile, break up the bread into small pieces, place in a bowl and pour the tomato juice over. Leave for some 5 minutes and then mix in the garlic, parsley, chilli and about 1½ tbsp of the remaining oil. Add the cooked aubergine flesh mixture and stir well, using a fork, which will more easily break up all the bits of bread. Taste and add salt to your liking.

Brush a baking sheet with a little olive oil and add the aubergine halves. Fill the halves with the stuffing, sprinkle with the dried breadcrumbs and drizzle with the remaining oil. Place the tray in the oven and bake for about 30 minutes until a light crust has formed on the top of the stuffing. Serve hot, but not straight from the oven, or at room temperature.

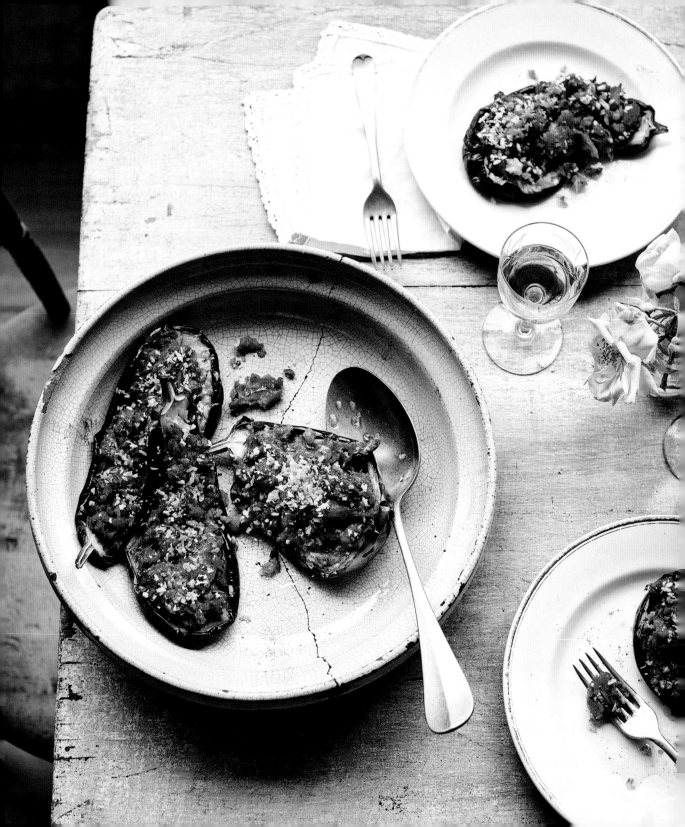

Pizzelle di Melanzane
Aubergine Pizzas

I love this dish – the similarity with pizza lies in its topping, which is piled on a slice of aubergine instead of on pizza dough. The aubergine slices can be roasted in a hot oven for 5 minutes or steamed as in this recipe.

Serves 4

3 aubergines (eggplant)
Extra virgin olive oil
250g/9oz buffalo mozzarella
Dried oregano

For the tomato sauce
1 x 125g/4oz can chopped tomatoes
2 tbsp extra virgin olive oil
1 garlic clove, crushed
1–2 pinches chilli (chili) flakes
2 pinches sea salt

Heat the oven to 180°C Fan/200°C/400°F/Gas Mark 6.

First make the tomato sauce. Put the tomatoes, oil, garlic, chilli and salt in a saucepan and cook, uncovered, over a lively heat for about 15 minutes, or until the oil has slightly separated from the tomatoes. Stir frequently. Taste and check the seasoning.

Remove the ends of the aubergines and wash and dry them. (You can keep these smaller ends for a ratatouille or a frittata.) Cut each aubergine into 1cm/½in slices, put the slices in a steamer and steam until tender. It is impossible to say how long this will take since it depends on the size of your steamer.

Brush a large baking sheet generously with some of the oil. Place the aubergine slices on the sheet, brush each one with some of the oil and sprinkle on a little salt.

Cut the mozzarella into 1cm/½in thick slices and place a slice over each aubergine slice. Top with a small teaspoon of tomato sauce and sprinkle with a little oregano. Place the tray in the oven and bake for 7–8 minutes. Serve hot.

Caponata di Melanzane
Aubergines in a Sweet and Sour Sauce

This Sicilian dish appears in many different versions throughout the island. It is based on a mixture of fried aubergine, celery, onion and tomato, to which artichokes or wild asparagus may be added. The mixture is sometimes garnished with small octopus, prawns or shrimps, small pieces of lobster or bottarga (dried mullet or tuna roe). The recipe here includes a small amount of chocolate. For an even richer *caponata*, a special sauce, called *salsa di San Bernardo*, is poured over it. This is made with sugar, vinegar, toasted almonds and dark chocolate: a sweet and sour sauce very much in the medieval style.

Serves 4

750g/1lb 10oz aubergines (eggplant)

Vegetable oil for frying

Sea salt

1 head of celery, inner stalks only,
*   coarse strings removed*

100ml/3 ½fl oz/7 tbsp olive oil

1 onion, very finely sliced

225g/8oz canned plum tomatoes,
*   drained and chopped*

Freshly ground black pepper

1 tbsp granulated sugar

6 tbsp white wine vinegar

1 tbsp grated dark chocolate (minimum
*   70% cocoa solids)*

4 tbsp capers, preferably in salt, rinsed

50g/1 ¾oz large green olives, stoned
*   (pitted) and quartered*

2 eggs, hard-boiled, to serve

Remove the ends of the aubergines and wash and dry them. (You can keep these smaller ends for a ratatouille or a frittata.) Cut the aubergines into 1cm/½in cubes.

Heat 2.5cm/1in vegetable oil in a frying pan. When the oil is hot, add a layer of aubergines and fry until golden brown on all sides. Drain on kitchen paper, sprinkling each batch lightly with salt. Repeat until all the aubergine is cooked.

Cut the celery into 1cm/½in cubes. Add the celery to the oil used for the aubergines and cook until golden and crisp. Drain on kitchen paper.

Pour the olive oil into a clean frying pan and add the onion. Sauté gently for about 10 minutes, until soft. Add the tomatoes and cook, stirring frequently, over a moderate heat for about 15 minutes. Season with salt and pepper to taste.

While the sauce is cooking, heat the sugar and vinegar in a small saucepan. Add the chocolate, capers and olives and simmer the mixture gently until the chocolate has melted. Add to the tomato sauce and cook for a further 5 minutes.

Mix the aubergines and celery into the tomato sauce. Stir and cook for 20 minutes, so that the flavours of the ingredients blend together. Pour the caponata into a serving dish and leave to cool.

Before serving, pass the eggs through the smallest holes of a food mill or push through a metal sieve over the caponata.

Patata
Potato

The potato arrived in Italy at the beginning of the 16th century, as the tomato did. But while the tomato soon became an emblem of Italian cooking, the potato never reached great popularity. This negative attitude in Italy gave this humble tuber the advantage that it was treated as a precious food in its own right and not just as a perfect accompaniment for mopping up the juices – we use bread for that. So forget about plain boiled potatoes and think about *patate trifolate*, *pasticcio di patate*, gnocchi, *insalata di patate*, *pure' di patate* and many other dishes.

Until the beginning of the 18th century, potatoes were considered food for animals or at best for peasants. They first became popular in France partly thanks to Antoine-Augustin Parmentier, who served them in his famous dish to Queen Marie-Antoinette. The queen loved it and Parmentier boasted that, in order to promote the potato, she pinned small bunches of potato flowers in her coiffure. The Italian scientist Alessandro Volta, better known for the invention of the electrical battery, allegedly was present at one of these court banquets. He, too, loved the humble tuber and began its cultivation in his estate near Lake Como, thus introducing it to the Italian aristocracy thereafter.

The potatoes of Lombardy are still excellent, as are those of Piedmont and Calabria, and potatoes are now cultivated everywhere in Italy. The best potatoes I ever had in my life were in a restaurant on the island of Ischia. They were simply boiled and served just with olive oil. I asked the patron where they came from and he told me they were grown in the volcanic soil on the slopes of Vesuvius, the best soil ever as the Romans well knew. All the wealthy Romans grew their produce around this part of Lazio and Campania.

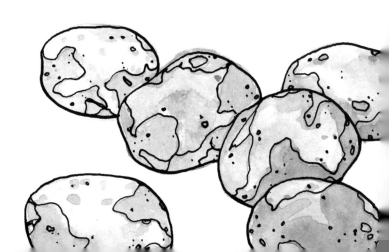

Patate al Diavolicchio
Warm Potato Salad with Chilli

This warm salad is a perfect accompaniment to cold meats, roast chicken or grilled fish. It is not a salad as such but this is the name that has stuck to the dish when it was first made by my grandson, Johnny. Johnny is a good cook with very discerning palate. He would make an excellent chef but is too lazy.

Serves 6

1kg/2lb 4oz waxy or salad potatoes
Salt
75ml/5 tbsp olive oil
2.5cm/1in piece fresh chilli (chili),
*   deseeded and very finely chopped*
2 garlic cloves, finely chopped

Cook the potatoes in their skins in boiling, salted water until just tender. Drain and peel as soon as they are cool enough to handle. Cool slightly, then cut into slices and sprinkle with salt.

Heat the oil in a pan. Add the chilli and garlic and fry for about 3 minutes until the garlic is lightly coloured. Take care not to burn the garlic or it will have a bitter taste. Pour the mixture over the potatoes. Toss gently together and serve warm.

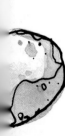

Bastoncini di Patate e Zucchine
Sautéed Potato and Courgette Sticks

Potatoes and courgettes go well together; their flavours seem to complement each other and they also look attractive together. I like courgettes tender, but if you prefer them slightly crunchy, add them to the potatoes a few minutes later. As for the herb added at the end, my favourite for this dish is dried oregano, but marjoram is also very good.

Serves 4

350g/12oz waxy potatoes

6 tbsp extra virgin olive oil

1 garlic clove, chopped

350g/12oz small courgettes (zucchini), but not baby ones

Sea salt and freshly ground black pepper

A generous sprinkling of dried oregano

Peel and wash the potatoes and cut them into sticks about 4cm/1½in long and 1cm/½in thick.

Heat the oil in a large frying pan, add the garlic and sauté for 1 minute. Add the potato sticks and sauté for 8–10 minutes, turning them over occasionally. Be careful that they do not scorch.

While the potatoes are cooking, wash and dry the courgettes and cut them into the same size sticks. When the potatoes are half done – about 10 minutes – add the courgette sticks, gradually, not all together, mixing after each addition. Season with salt and pepper and cook until the vegetables are done. Sprinkle with the oregano, taste and adjust the seasoning.

Patate Trifolate
Sautéed Potatoes with Parsley and Garlic

Trifolato means cooked in butter and oil with garlic and parsley, and many vegetables, such as mushrooms, courgettes, aubergines and carrots, are cooked this way. It is in fact very easy, but it requires a watchful eye. You go away for 5 minutes and you come back to a blackened bottom. Still, the dish does not take long to cook.

Serves 4

750g/1lb 10oz waxy potatoes
2 garlic cloves, bruised
25g/1oz/2 tbsp unsalted butter
3 tbsp olive oil
25g/1oz/1 cup flat leaf parsley,
    chopped
Sea salt and freshly ground black
    pepper

Peel and wash the potatoes. Cut them into small cubes of about 2cm/¾in.

Thread the garlic cloves with a wooden stick. This will make it easier to remove the garlic before serving. However, if you prefer a stronger garlic flavour, chop the cloves and leave them in.

Heat the butter and the oil with half the parsley and the garlic in a large sauté pan and when hot gradually add the potatoes, mixing well after each addition. Cook over a lively heat for about 8 minutes, mixing frequently. Discard the garlic and add about 4–5 tablespoons of hot water.

Stir, cover the pan and cook over a low heat until the potatoes are tender, about 20–25 minutes. Stir occasionally using a fork rather than a spoon, because a fork is less likely to break the potatoes. If the potatoes begin to stick to the bottom of the pan, add a little more hot water. Halfway through the cooking, season with salt – potatoes are more likely to break up if you add the salt at the beginning of the cooking.

When the potatoes are tender, season with pepper, check the salt and sprinkle with the remaining parsley before serving.

Gattò di Patate
Potato Cake with Mozzarella and Prosciutto

You can serve this *gattò* hot or warm as a first course, or as a second course after a soup.

Serves 4

850g/1lb 14oz floury (starchy)
  potatoes

100ml/3½fl oz/scant ½ cup full-fat
  (whole) milk

75g/2¾oz/5 tbsp unsalted butter

Sea salt and freshly ground black
  pepper

A small grating of nutmeg

8 tbsp freshly grated Parmesan

2 large (US extra-large) eggs

1 large (US extra-large) egg yolk

200g/7oz mozzarella cheese, cut into
  slices

75g/2¾oz prosciutto, not too thinly
  sliced

75g/2¾oz mortadella or salami, sliced

For the tin and topping

20g/¾oz/1½ tbsp unsalted butter

4–5 tbsp dried breadcrumbs

Scrub the potatoes and cook them in their skins in plenty of water until you can easily pierce through to the middle with the point of a small knife.

Meanwhile, heat the oven to 180°C Fan/200°C/400°F/Gas Mark 6. Butter a 20cm/8in diameter springform cake tin and coat the surface with some of the breadcrumbs. Shake out any excess crumbs.

Drain the potatoes and peel them as soon as they are cool enough to handle. Pass them through a food mill or potato ricer to make a purée, letting it fall into the pan in which the potatoes were cooked.

Heat the milk and add to the purée with the butter. Beat well and then add ½ tsp of salt, pepper to taste, nutmeg and the Parmesan. Mix well, add the eggs and egg yolk and mix again very thoroughly. Spoon half the potato mixture into the prepared tin, cover with the mozzarella, prosciutto and mortadella, then spoon the rest of the purée over the top. Dot with a little butter and sprinkle very lightly with the remaining breadcrumbs.

Bake for 20–30 minutes, until the *gattò* is brown on top and hot in the middle (test by inserting a small knife into the middle and then bringing it to your lip – it should feel hot). If it is still a bit pale, flash it under the grill. Allow the *gattò* to stand for 10 minutes before serving.

Gnocchi di Patate
Potato Gnocchi

Of all the different types of gnocchi, these are the most popular. They might be popular, but they are not so easy to make, as so much depends on the variety of the potatoes. The best potatoes to use are floury ones and try to get them all more or less the same size. I prefer gnocchi made without egg, the gnocchi of northern Italy, which are light and fluffy.

The most popular sauces for potato gnocchi are a butter sauce, such as the butter and sage dressing used for the *Gnocchi di Barbabietola* or Beetroot Gnocchi (see page 21), a simple tomato sauce or some *Pesto* or Basil Sauce (see page 196).

Serves 4–6

1kg/2lb 4oz floury (starchy) potatoes

175–200g/6–7oz/1 1/3–1 1/2 cups flour

Sea salt

Freshly grated Parmesan to serve

Cook the potatoes in their skins in plenty of water. When the point of a knife can be pushed through to the middle, the potatoes are ready. Drain and peel them as soon as they are cool enough to handle. Pass them through a food mill or potato ricer while still hot straight on to your work surface.

Add 2 tsp of salt and most of the flour to the mashed potatoes and knead into a smooth mixture. Some potatoes need more flour than others, so it is best not to add all the flour at once. Stop adding flour when the dough becomes soft and smooth but still sticky. Shape the dough into a ball, wrap in clingfilm and leave to rest for half an hour – it does not matter if you leave it longer.

To make the gnocchi, pinch a handful of dough from the ball and shape it into a sausage about 2.5cm/1in thick. Cut the sausage into 2cm/¾in chunks. Repeat with the rest of the dough. Now you can leave your gnocchi as they are – soft little pillows – or you can give them the characteristic grooves. The grooves are there for a reason: for thinning out the gnocchi and for trapping more dressing. Flip each gnocco against the floured prongs of a fork, without dragging it hard. Some cooks flip the gnocchi toward the handle of the fork, others, like I do, flip them toward the points of the prong. You find your favourite way.

Put a large saucepan of water on the heat. When the water is boiling fast, add 2 tbsp of salt and drop in about one-third of the gnocchi. The gnocchi will sink to the bottom of the pan, then give them a gentle stir and they will soon begin to float. Count to 20 and then start lifting them out of the water with a slotted spoon. Quickly pat them dry with kitchen paper and transfer them to a heated dish. Dress each cooked batch with a little of the sauce you are using. When all the gnocchi are cooked, pour the remaining sauce over and serve with plenty of grated Parmesan cheese.

Croquettes di Patate al Forno
Baked Potato Cakes

The traditional way to cook croquettes in Italy is to fry them in butter and oil. I love fried foods, but I know it is not an easy method of cooking. Not only that, it is also rather a boring one, since you have to do it at the last minute. So in this recipe I decided to bake the croquettes instead of frying them. It is far easier and they taste just as good.

Buy potatoes all the same size, if you can.

Serves 4

750g/1lb 10oz floury (starchy)
    potatoes
Sea salt
125g/4½oz/9 tbsp unsalted butter,
    cut into small pieces
1 egg, gently beaten
3 tbsp freshly grated Parmesan
Freshly ground black pepper

Scrub the potatoes, put them in a saucepan, cover with water and bring to the boil. Add 1 tbsp of salt and simmer until tender when you prick them with the point of a knife. Drain and peel them as soon as they are cool enough to handle.

Heat the oven to 200°C Fan/220°C/425°F/Gas Mark 7.

Pass the potatoes through a food mill or potato ricer, letting the purée fall into a bowl. Add 100g/3½oz/scant ½ cup of the butter, the egg, cheese and pepper. Mix well and then taste and adjust the salt.

Melt the remaining butter in a small saucepan and, when melted, use some of it to lightly brush a baking sheet. Divide the purée into lumps about the size of a tennis ball and shape them like an egg. Place on the sheet and brush the croquettes with melted butter. Place the sheet in the oven and bake for 20 minutes, until the potato cakes are golden. Remove from the oven and leave to rest for 2–3 minutes before serving.

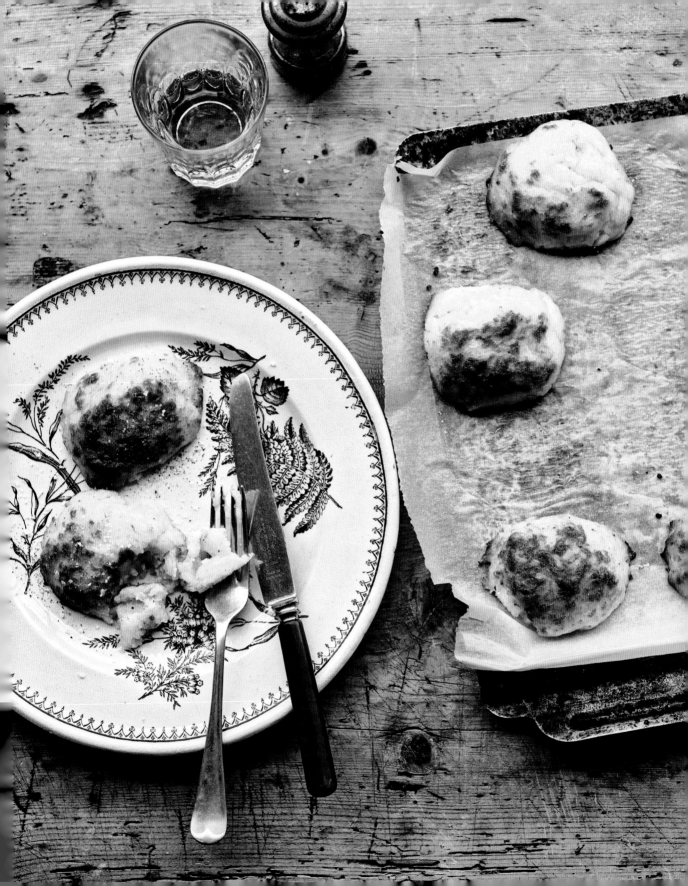

Pure' di Patate
Mashed Potatoes

In Italy mashed potatoes are a dish in their own right, not just an accompaniment to meat or fish. The potatoes should be the floury variety because they remain more fluffy when mashed. This is the way our wonderful cook, Maria, used to make *pure'di patate* in our kitchen in pre-war Milan. I still make it like that in my post-war kitchen looking out on the Dorset hills. And when I eat it I travel back to those times, as I always do when eating dishes I used to eat in my childhood. Nothing is more nostalgic than food – except for maybe music.

Try to buy potatoes all the same size.

Serves 4

1kg/2lb 4oz floury (starchy) potatoes
1 shallot, very finely chopped
75g/2¾oz/5 tbsp unsalted butter
100–150ml/3½–5fl oz/scant
   ½–⅔ cup full fat (whole) milk
2 tbsp freshly grated Parmesan
2 tbsp chopped flat leaf parsley
Sea salt and freshly ground black
   pepper

Scrub the potatoes and put them in a large saucepan. Cover with cold water, add 1 tbsp of salt and bring to the boil. Cook at a gentle simmer until the potatoes can easily be pierced by the point of a knife, which will take at least 20 minutes. Drain and, as soon as they are cool enough to handle, peel them – it is easier to peel them while they are still hot. Pass the potatoes through a food mill or potato ricer, letting the purée fall into a bowl.

Add the shallot and butter to a sauté pan and cook until just turning gold. Mix in the potato purée and turn it over and over to absorb all the butter. Heat the milk in a small saucepan until just coming up to the boil and slowly add to the purée. Add the milk gradually and stop when the purée is soft but not too much so. It is impossible to give the right quantity because it depends on the variety of potato. Mix in the cheese and parsley and add salt and pepper to taste.

Polpettone di Zucchine
Potato and Courgette Bake

In Liguria vegetables are cooked in many different ways. Very often they are the main dish of the meal and this is a good example. You really cannot eat much else after this!

Serves 6

500g/1lb 2oz floury (starchy) potatoes, all the same size

100ml/3½fl oz/7 tbsp olive oil

1 red onion, finely chopped

2 garlic cloves, finely chopped

750g/1lb 10oz courgettes (zucchini)

25g/1oz/1 cup flat leaf parsley, chopped

4 eggs

5 tbsp freshly grated Parmesan

2 tsp dried oregano

A grating of nutmeg

Dried breadcrumbs

Sea salt and freshly ground black pepper

Scrub the potatoes, put them in a saucepan, cover with water and cook them until tender. Drain and peel them as soon as you can handle them – it is easier to remove the skins when the potatoes are still hot. Pass them through a food mill or potato ricer into a large bowl – a food processor is not suitable because it will not aerate the potato.

While the potatoes are cooking, heat 4 tbsp of the oil in a large sauté pan. When hot, add the onion, garlic and 1 tsp of salt and sauté gently for 5 minutes, stirring occasionally.

Heat the oven to 160°C Fan/180°C/350°F/Gas Mark 4.

Wash and dry the courgettes and cut them into 3mm/⅛in rounds as thick as a pound coin. Add the courgettes to the onion and sauté them for 5 minutes, turning them over frequently so all the rounds become coated in oil. Add the parsley, 2–3 tbsp of hot water and salt and pepper to taste, cover the pan and continue cooking over a low heat for about 15 minutes until the courgettes are done. Do not forget to turn them over every now and then. Add a little more hot water if the courgettes start to stick to the bottom of the pan. When they are done, scoop them with their juices into the bowl with the potatoes. Mix well.

Lightly beat the eggs together, mix in the Parmesan, oregano, nutmeg and salt and pepper and then add the mixture to the vegetable purée. Mix thoroughly.

Oil an ovenproof dish and lightly sprinkle with some breadcrumbs. Spoon in the potato and courgette mixture. Sprinkle some breadcrumbs over the top and dribble with the remaining oil. Bake for 30 minutes. Remove from the oven and leave to rest for a few minutes before serving. You can also serve it at room temperature.

Peperone
Pepper

Peppers, both sweet and chilli peppers, arrived from the New World at the beginning of the 16th century, along with potatoes and tomatoes. As with these two vegetables, they belong to the solanum or nightshade family so were thought to be poisonous and they took quite a time to become popular. Vincenzo Corrado, writing at the end of the 18th century, described them as 'vulgar food for the peasants' and it was only in the 19th century that peppers became a popular vegetable. It may well be that the peppers cultivated then were still very hot and thus were considered 'vulgar' food. Artusi writing at the end of the 19th century has no recipe for peppers, while Ada Boni, some 50 years later, has 17 recipes for peppers of which seven are for stuffed peppers. I particularly like the sound of her peppers stuffed with boiled small octopus and calameretti. I must try it.

The peppers grown in Italy are the sweetest in the world and, at the same time, also those with the strongest capsicum flavour, their peculiar but necessary flavour. The best peppers are grown on the gentle hills between southern Piedmont and Lombardy and, as for many other vegetables, around the city of Naples.

Peppers come in different shapes – long and pointed or squat and square – and different colours, from ivory to purple, the most common being the green, red and yellow. The green are the least sweet of the lot and more suitable to cooking than eating raw. The easiest way to serve grilled peppers is dress them with the best olive oil, mashed preserved anchovies, salt and pepper to taste, and a touch of garlic.

Peppers lend themselves to being stuffed with many different ingredients, from rice to meat and pasta or just simply breadcrumbs, parsley and garlic – the basic stuffing of *cucina povera*. Of all the pepper dishes, the most famous is *peperonata*, the classic accompaniment to *bollito misto* – boiled meats – both in Piedmont and in Lombardy. This reminds me that the best peperonata I have ever had was in Asti at the table of a friend Carlo, who was the managing director of the Sacla company, famous for its ready-made pesto sauce. The peperonata, lovingly cooked by Carlo himself, accompanied a *gran bollito misto* containing also the *testina* (calf's head) and the *piedini* (calf's trotters).

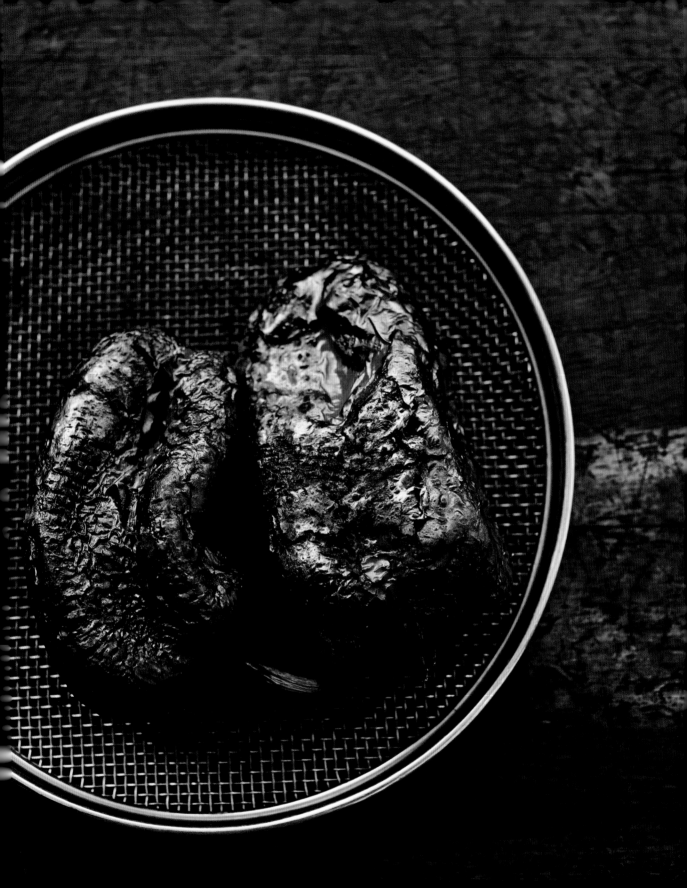

Peperoni alla Siciliana
Grilled Peppers with Anchovies, Olives and Capers

I love grilled peppers in every way, but this is a particularly good recipe, thanks to the vinegary onion sauce in which they are finished off.

For this dish round peppers, not the long ones, are better because they have a thicker skin.

Serves 4

5 red and yellow round peppers (bell
    peppers)

4 tbsp extra virgin olive oil

1 red onion, finely sliced

Sea salt

2 garlic cloves, chopped

1 tsp Marigold vegetable bouillon
    powder

2 tbsp balsamic vinegar

1 tbsp caster (granulated) sugar

Freshly ground black pepper

1 tbsp dried oregano

16 black olives, stoned (pitted) and cut
    into strips

6 anchovy fillets, drained, or
    3 preserved anchovies, cleaned and
    rinsed

2 tbsp small capers, rinsed

First you need to grill the peppers. The best way to do this is directly over a flame, rather than under a grill. Put a wire rack on the gas ring and then place one or two peppers straight on it and leave them until the skin is black. Turn the peppers over and burn another side of the pepper and continue until the whole pepper is blackish. Be careful not to leave the pepper too long in the same position or it will burn through the pulp as well and you will have a hole. Repeat with the remaining peppers. If you do not have a direct flame, put the peppers under the grill and turn them over and over until they are charred all over.

Remove the skins using your hands or a small knife. Don't wash the peppers because you will wash away their juices. Wipe the peppers clean with damp kitchen paper, cut them in half, then in quarters and remove the cores and seeds. Now cut each quarter vertically into about 2cm/¾in strips. Now the peppers are ready to be used.

Put the oil and the onion in a frying pan, sprinkle with salt and add 2 tbsp of water. Cook gently for about 15 minutes, stirring frequently and then add the garlic and continue cooking for about 40 minutes until the onion is like a golden mush.

Mix in the peppers, the bouillon powder, vinegar, sugar and pepper to taste and cook over a very low heat for some 20 minutes, turning the whole thing over now and then. If the mixture gets too dry, add a couple of tablespoons of hot water. Add the oregano, olives, anchovies and capers, mix well and continue cooking, always over a low heat, for 10 minutes. Serve warm or at room temperature with plenty of crusty bread.

Peperoni all'Aceto
Peppers in a Vinegary Sauce

I have made these peppers in vinegar for many years. But recently I have changed from stewing them directly on the heat to baking them in the oven and this new method of cooking thm makes it altogether easier.

Serves 4

6 large peppers (bell peppers)

5 tbsp extra virgin olive oil

2 tbsp wine vinegar

1 tbsp balsamic vinegar

1 tbsp dried oregano

6 garlic cloves, bruised

Sea salt and freshly ground black
*   pepper*

Wash the peppers, cut them in quarters and remove the cores and seeds. Put them in a big bowl.

In a small bowl, mix together the oil, the two vinegars, oregano, salt and a good grinding of peppers. Pour this *salsina* over the peppers and mix well using your hands. Add the bruised garlic cloves and, if you have time, leave them to marinate for at least 30 minutes – the longer the better.

Toward the end of the marinating time, heat the oven to 180°C Fan/ 200°C/400°F/Gas Mark 6.

Spread the peppers on a baking sheet and add all the juices. Bake for 10–12 minutes. The peppers will be slightly charred on the outside and still crunchy. These peppers are lovely cold, but you can also eat them warm.

Peperoni alla Piemontese
Roasted Peppers with Hard-Boiled Eggs

This is a classic Piedmontese dish which appears on every antipasto trolley in every restaurant in northern Italy and often also in the south. It is certainly one of the most appetizing ways to eat peppers. The only catch is that the peppers should be fat and juicy so that, when the skins are removed, there is still a lot of pulp to sink one's teeth into. Try to buy heavy peppers, as the heavier they are the thicker the pulp.

Serves 4

4–5 red and yellow peppers (bell peppers)

4 hard-boiled eggs, shelled

50g/1 ¾oz anchovy fillets preserved in olive oil, drained

1 garlic clove

25g/1oz/1 cup flat leaf parsley

6 tbsp extra virgin olive oil

1 tbsp wine vinegar, balsamic is good here

2–3 tbsp small capers, rinsed

Sea salt and freshly ground black pepper

First you need to grill the peppers. The best way to do this is directly over a flame, rather than under a grill. Put a wire rack on the gas ring and then place one or two peppers straight on it and leave them until the skin is black. Turn the peppers over and burn another side of the pepper and continue until the whole pepper is blackish. Be careful not to leave the pepper too long in the same position or it will burn through the pulp as well and you will have a hole. Repeat with the remaining peppers. If you do not have a direct flame, put the peppers under the grill and turn them over and over until they are charred all over.

Remove the skins using your hands or a small knife. Don't wash the peppers because you will wash away their juices. Wipe the peppers clean with damp kitchen paper, cut them in half and remove the cores and seeds.

Cut the pepper halves into strips and lay the strips in a large dish or on individual plates. I always prefer a large dish because it allows my guests or family to help themselves to the amount they want.

Cut the hard-boiled eggs in half and place them here and there on the peppers. Divide the anchovy fillets in two lengthwise and do the same.

Cut the garlic in half and remove the inside greenish germ, if present, and chop the garlic together with the parsley and put in a bowl. Gradually pour in the oil and the vinegar, while beating gently with a fork. Season with salt – not much because of the anchovies – and pepper and spoon the *salsina* over the peppers. Scatter with the capers. Leave the dish to rest for around 30 minutes before serving.

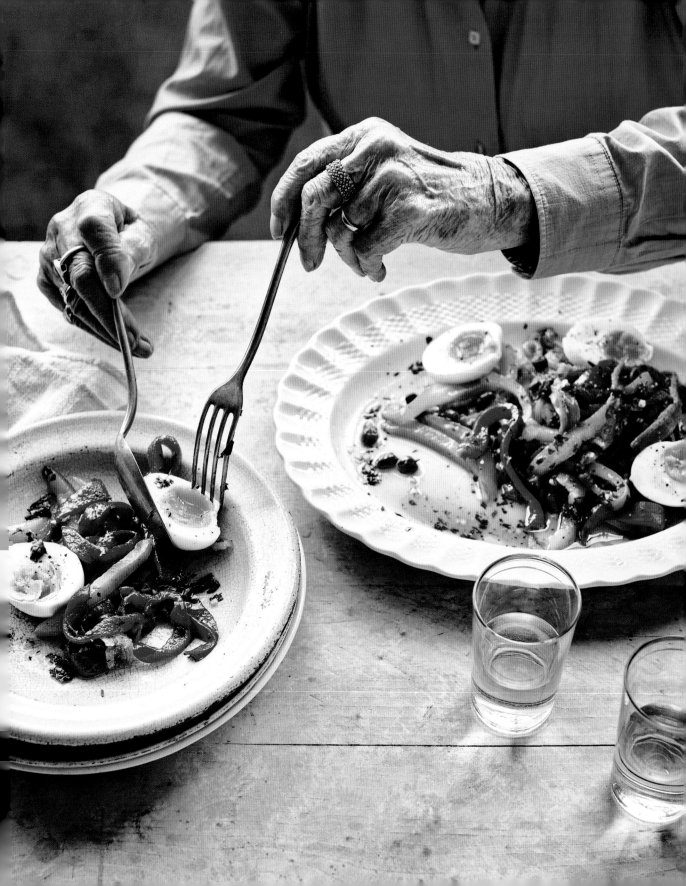

Peperoni Ripieni di Formaggio di Capra e Pesto
Peppers Stuffed with Goat's Cheese and Pesto

My mother used to make these peppers when she prepared a dish of stuffed vegetables in the summer. Sometimes she served them alongside roasted aubergine halves and tomatoes stuffed with the same ingredients, while in the autumn the aubergines would be replaced by her delicious *Scodelle di Cipolle Ripiene* or Onions Stuffed with Tuna (see page 65) and stuffed porcini caps. Different seasons, different vegetables, different stuffing. Of all the different stuffings the most common was a simple one made with breadcrumbs, parsley and garlic, hardly a stuffing, more of a dressing really.

Serves 4

4 large yellow and red peppers (bell peppers)

3 tbsp extra virgin olive oil

2 garlic cloves, crushed

100g/3½oz soft goat's cheese

1 tbsp yogurt

1 tbsp basil pesto

A few fresh basil leaves

Sea salt and freshly ground black pepper

Fresh wild rocket (arugula), optional

First you need to grill the peppers. The best way to do this is directly over a flame, rather than under a grill. Put a wire rack on the gas ring and then place one or two peppers straight on it and leave them until the skin is black. Turn the peppers over and burn another side of the pepper and continue until the whole pepper is blackish. Be careful not to leave the pepper too long in the same position or it will burn through the pulp as well and you will have a hole. Repeat with the remaining peppers. If you do not have a direct flame, put the peppers under the grill and turn them over and over until they are charred all over.

Remove the skins using your hands or a small knife. Don't wash the peppers because you will wash away their juices. Wipe the peppers clean with damp kitchen paper, cut them in half and remove the cores and seeds.

Put the peppers in a dish, dress them with 2 tbsp of the oil, scatter the garlic on top and season with salt and pepper. Leave to absorb the flavours for at least 1 hour.

Put the cheese in a bowl, add the yogurt and the pesto and mix together well. It is more efficient to do this with a fork than with a spoon. Now add the remaining oil and a good grinding of pepper. Taste and check the salt.

Place 2 pepper halves on each plate and fill each half with the mixture. Sprinkle the basil leaves over the top and serve. I like to place the peppers on a cushion of rocket lightly 'christened' with some extra virgin olive oil and a touch of salt.

Peperonata
Pepper and Tomato Ratatouille

When I was a child in Milan, *peperonata* always appeared on our table on Mondays to accompany the big dish of *lesso* (boiled beef) of *bollito misto*, a dish of mixed boiled meats. The *lesso* consisted of one large piece of beef, while *bollito misto* was a big platter of beef, half a chicken, fresh tongue and calf's jowl, surrounded by boiled potatoes, boiled carrots, boiled onions and, finally, *peperonata*, whose bright red, yellow and green colours brought life – and flavour – to a dish of a subdued nature. But you don't need to serve *peperonata* just with boiled meats. I love it also with roast pork, steak or roast chicken. And if you have any left over, it makes a wonderful spaghetti sauce.

Buy large square peppers which are more meaty than the long, pointed ones.

Serves 4–6

1kg/2lb 4oz large peppers (bell peppers), red, yellow and green
6 tbsp extra virgin olive oil
2 onions, sliced
1 small red chilli (chili)
2 garlic cloves, chopped
750g/1lb 10oz ripe tomatoes, peeled and coarsely chopped
1 tbsp brown sugar
2 tbsp balsamic vinegar
25g/1oz/1 cup flat leaf parsley, chopped
Sea salt and freshly ground black pepper

Heat the oven to 160°C Fan/180°C/350°F/Gas Mark 4.

Wash and dry the peppers. Cut them vertically in half and then in quarters. Remove and discard all the cores and seeds and cut them lengthwise into roughly 1cm/½in strips.

Heat the oil in a large sauté pan and when hot add the onions with a pinch or two of salt and cook over a medium heat until soft. Stir frequently so that the onion becomes soft and golden but not brown.

Remove the seeds and core of the hot chilli, cut into very small bits and add to the onions together with the garlic. Continue cooking for a further minute and then add the peppers and cook for about 10 minutes over a lively heat, stirring frequently so that the peppers become coated in the oil.

Mix in the tomatoes with all their juices, bring the dish to a simmer and cook for about 15 minutes to evaporate some of the liquid. Add the sugar and allow it to caramelize a little while you gently stir and then add the vinegar. Mix well, season to taste and continue cooking until the peppers are soft – the peppers in *peperonata* should be quite soft, not al dente, and this will take a further 45 minutes–1 hour. Then sprinkle the top with the chopped parsley and serve either hot, warm or at room temperature.

Piselli
Peas

Peas are one of the most popular vegetables. I wonder if it is because they have a certain amount of sweetness and because they freeze so well – frozen peas are a good standby in any freezer. Canned peas are widely used in Italian homes.

Peas have been eaten since time immemorial. They originally came from Mesopotamia – as did most of the early European vegetables – and by Roman times they were a common food. These were not the peas we are used to. They were coarser, both in taste and in texture, and were usually dried. The variety of peas we now know was developed in Italy and by the 16th century they were a well-established food. These were the peas that, according to legend, were introduced to France by Caterina de' Medici, who served them at her wedding to Henry II in 1530. I find the story pretty unlikely as I believe peas were already known in France well before the 16th century.

The best peas come fresh in pods from 8–10cm/3¼–4in long. The pods should be bright green and crisp and look well filled but not bulging. If the pods are unblemished and fresh-looking you can use them to make stock and puréed pods are used in the famous recipe from Veneto *risi e bisi*.

If you buy fresh peas in their pods you need to allow 1kg/2lb 4oz to give approximately 500g/1lb 2oz shelled weight.

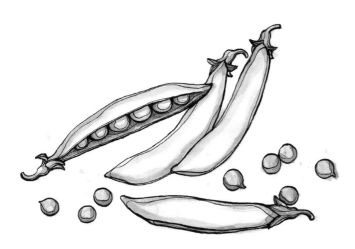

Piselli al Prosciutto
Peas with Prosciutto

Peas and prosciutto are a very good combination of flavours, the prosciutto lending the peas just the right amount of bite.

You need to buy the prosciutto in thick slices of about 5mm/¼in. The prosciutto sold already sliced in plastic envelopes is no good for this recipe.

Serves 4

1kg/2lb 4oz fresh peas in their pods or
500g/1lb 2oz shelled fresh peas or
frozen peas, thawed and drained
1 leek
40g/1½oz/3 tbsp unsalted butter, cut
into small pieces
100g/3½oz prosciutto
Sea salt and freshly ground black
pepper

Shell the peas if you are using fresh ones.

For this recipe you need only the white part of a medium size leek (keep the green leaves for a soup). Cut the leek into thin rings and wash thoroughly in a bowl of cold water until there is no sand left at the bottom of the bowl.

Drain and put the leek rings in a sauté pan together with the butter. Gently sauté for a few minutes and then add the peas. Gently stir them around in the butter and leek *soffritto* for a minute or two and then add enough water to almost cover them. Cook, uncovered, over a low heat until the peas are done to your liking.

While the peas are cooking, cut the prosciutto into short strips, about 5cm/2in long. When the peas are done and all the liquid has been absorbed, mix in the prosciutto and add salt and pepper to taste. Serve hot.

Piselli al Dragoncello
Peas with Tarragon

Tarragon is one of the many herbs used in Tuscan cooking, although it appears very seldom in the cooking of other regions of Italy. This is a recipe from Siena.

Serves 4

1kg/2lb 4oz fresh peas in their pods or 500g/1lb 2oz shelled fresh peas or frozen peas, thawed and drained

4 tbsp olive oil

1 tsp caster (granulated) sugar

1 small shallot, very finely chopped

2 sprigs of tarragon, about 10cm/4in long

Sea salt and freshly ground black pepper

Shell the peas if you are using fresh ones. Put the peas in a saucepan and add enough hot water to come 5mm/¼in up the side of the pan. Add the remaining ingredients and bring to a gentle boil. Cover the pan and cook until the peas are tender, which depends on the quality and size of the peas, whether fresh or frozen, and on how you like them cooked – for instance, I like them cooked softer than al dente.

If there is still too much liquid in the saucepan when the peas are ready, remove the peas with a slotted spoon and boil briskly for the liquid to reduce. Taste and check the seasoning.

Cooked this way, peas make a delicious accompaniment to roast chicken, frittata or even to baked fish, such as sea bass.

Piselli e Funghetti al Sapor di Maggiorana
Peas and Mushrooms with Marjoram

Peas are a good accompaniment to most meat and fish dishes. Their delicate flavour blends easily with the main ingredient. In this recipe their flavour is enhanced by a few sliced mushrooms and some fresh marjoram. Marjoram is an easy herb to grow and mine is taking over one of the borders in my garden.

Serves 4–6

700g/1lb 9oz fresh peas in their pods
*   or 300g/10½oz shelled fresh peas*
*   or frozen peas, thawed and drained*
50g/1¾oz/4 tbsp unsalted butter
1 shallot, very finely chopped
Sea salt
250g/9oz button mushrooms, thickly
*   sliced*
150ml/5fl oz/⅔ cup vegetable stock
Freshly ground black pepper
1 tbsp chopped marjoram leaves

Shell the peas if you are using fresh ones.

Heat the butter in a pan and when the froth has subsided, add the shallot and a pinch of salt. Sauté for 2 minutes and then add the mushrooms. Cook for 5 minutes, turning the mushrooms over frequently.

Add the stock and peas and cook until they are tender. If there is still too much liquid in the pan when the peas are done, fish the vegetables out with a slotted spoon and keep warm in a low oven while you reduce the liquid over a high heat to a syrupy consistency. Spoon the sauce over the peas and mushrooms, season with salt and pepper to taste and sprinkle with the marjoram leaves.

133

Stracciatella Marchigiana
Stracciatella with Peas

You may have eaten *stracciatella*, the well known soup from Rome made with chicken stock, eggs, semolina and a lot of Parmesan cheese. In Le Marche, the region east of Rome, they add some peas and lemon rind and I prefer this variation.

Serves 4

3 eggs

3 tbsp semolina

4 tbsp freshly grated Parmesan

Sea salt and freshly ground black
    pepper

Grated rind of 1 unwaxed lemon

1.2 litres/2 pints/5 cups chicken or
    vegetable stock

200g/7oz shelled fresh peas or frozen
    peas, thawed and drained

25g/1oz/1 cup marjoram leaves,
    chopped

Beat the eggs lightly in a heatproof bowl and gradually add the semolina and the Parmesan. Season with salt and pepper and add half the grated lemon rind.

Add the stock to a saucepan and heat to simmering point. Pour one ladleful of the stock over the egg mixture. Beat gently and pour the mixture back into the simmering stock. Beat for 1–2 minutes and then add the peas and the remaining lemon rind. Cook until the peas are done to your liking.

Ladle the soup into individual bowls and sprinkle with a few marjoram leaves.

Vellutata di piselli e pere
Pea and Pear Soup

The adjective *vellutata* comes from the word *velluto*, which means 'velvet' and is used to describe smooth, puréed soups. I doubt this is a typical Italian soup but it was given to me by my Italian friend Myriam, who learnt it from her mother who, in her turn, used to make this soup with the pears which grew in her garden on Lake Orta in Piedmont. Whatever its origins, it is well worth making.

Serves 4

1 onion, very finely sliced

2 tbsp olive oil

30g/1oz/2 tbsp unsalted butter

Sea salt

12 mint leaves, torn

2 ripe pears, peeled and cut into small pieces

500g/1lb 2oz frozen peas

1 litre/1¾ pints/4 cups chicken stock

Freshly ground black pepper

Double (heavy) cream, optional

Gently sauté the onion, together with a pinch of salt and half the torn mint leaves, in the oil and butter for 8–10 minutes, stirring very frequently. The onion should become soft, not golden.

Add the pear to the onion. Sauté for 1 minute and then add the frozen peas with all their ice attached. Mix well and add the stock. Bring to the boil and simmer for 25 minutes. Blend the soup with a stick blender or in a liquidizer and season with salt and pepper to taste.

Ladle the soup into individual bowls, sprinkle with the remaining mint leaves and drop a blob of cream in the middle of each bowl, if you want.

Pomodoro
Tomato

It is difficult to imagine what Italian cooking was like before the arrival of this red fruit. The odd thing is that when the tomato first arrived from Central America at the beginning of the 16th century, it was looked upon with suspicion and distaste. However, apparently it was not the tomato we know now. It was a small, golden fruit – hence its name of *pomodoro* (golden apple) – but also quite acidic and mouth puckering. The strain of tomato as we know it now was successfully developed in Campania, in the fertile volcanic soil around Mount Vesuvius. The tomatoes from here are still considered among the best. And tomatoes are now the most widespread crop of Puglia, Sicily, Emilia-Romagna and Sardinia.

In the 16th century tomatoes were used on their branches mostly for table decorations, as some paintings of that period testify. The 17th-century cookery writer Antonio Latini cooks tomatoes with fresh chilli and gives recipes for a tomato sauce which is really the precursor of all tomato sauces. But it is not until the late 19th century that tomato sauce became very popular – in Naples the street vendors of *maccheroni* combined the two. They piled up the spaghetti on a dish and covered it with a ladleful of red sauce.

The 19th-century cook Artusi wrote the first recipe for stuffed tomatoes, his stuffing consisting of a *soffritto* of onion, mushrooms and parsley mixed with breadcrumbs, egg and cheese. They are then lavishly covered with melted butter (Artusi was a lover of butter rather than oil, but you can use oil, although the final flavour would be different) and braised in a covered pot in a moderate oven for a good hour.

Nowadays tomatoes are an intrinsic part of the Italian cookery scene, even sometimes too much so, as they appear in dishes that are better – or at least as good – without tomatoes, such as spaghetti with clams, *ossobuchi* or braised beef. Having said so, a salad of really good tomatoes cut in wedges, sprinkled with sea salt and dressed with good olive oil and maybe a touch of vinegar or lemon juice is hard to beat, as is a steaming dish of *spaghetti alla pomarola* to give it the authentic Neapolitan name. Fresh tomatoes are often replaced in cooking by canned tomatoes or passata (sieved tomatoes with a sauce-like consistency).

Pomodorini Arrostiti
Roasted Cherry Tomatoes

This is hardly a recipe but I just want to tell you how quick and easy it is to roast a few tomatoes, a process that brings out their flavour.

Heat the oven to 180°C Fan/200°C/400°F/Gas Mark 6.

Cut the tomatoes in half and put them in a large bowl. Pour in a good drizzle of extra virgin olive oil and season with salt and pepper. Mix well, but gently so as not to break them. Place on a baking sheet and roast for 5–7 minutes, until just slightly wrinkled and bubbling.

Bruschetta col Pomodoro
Tomato Bruschetta

This bruschetta is worth making only with very good tomatoes with thin skins, since they should not be peeled.

Serves 4
6 ripe tomatoes
Sea salt
1 ciabatta
2 garlic cloves, cut in half
6 tbsp extra virgin olive oil
12 basil leaves, torn

Cut the tomatoes in half and then cut away and discard the cores. Cut the tomatoes into small cubes and season with salt. Leave them on one side for about 30 minutes.

Cut the ciabatta diagonally into 1cm/½in thick slices. Score each slice lightly with the point of a small knife, rub with the garlic on both sides, moisten with some olive oil and place them on a grill or barbecue rack. Grill until charred on both sides.

Place a few pieces of tomatoes on each slice, dress with the remaining oil and scatter a few pieces of basil on top.

Panzanella
Tomato, Spring Onion, Cucumber and Crouton Salad

The motherland of *panzanella* is Tuscany, whose cuisine is one of the most *povera* of all *cucine povere* of Italy and, as such, bread is one of its main ingredients. Until recently in Italy only the rich could afford to buy meat and fish and the *cucina povera* (cooking of the poor) as practised by the peasant classes had to use whatever was available in the kitchen or farm or the vegetables grown in their back gardens. My version of *panzanella* is a gentrified version of the original. I use *crostini* because I find it difficult to find the right bread when not in Italy and also because I prefer to munch something slightly cracking than something mushy.

Serves 4

½ large cucumber

250g/9oz cherry tomatoes

6 spring onions (scallions)

1 garlic clove

200g/7oz crostini (see page 199)

2 tbsp wine vinegar

5 tbsp extra virgin olive oil

Sea salt and freshly ground black pepper

12 fresh basil leaves, torn into coarse pieces

Wash the cucumber and use a potato peeler to shave the skin off in strips so that at the end you have a dark and pale green striped cucumber. Cut into slices and put into a salad bowl.

Wash the tomatoes and cut in half and add to the bowl. I don't peel the cherry tomatoes for this salad, but if you object to their skins, peel them by immersing them in boiling water for 30 seconds and then rinse them under cold running water.

Cut off the green foliage and roots of the spring onions. Wash and cut them in slices. Add to the bowl. Remove the germ from the garlic clove if necessary, chop and add to the bowl. Now mix in the crostini.

Pour the vinegar over the salad, stir and then pour in the oil. Season with salt and a good grinding of pepper and mix very thoroughly. Taste and check the seasoning.

Put the salad in the refrigerator for about 30 minutes; the salad is better slightly cold. Scatter the basil leaves over the top before serving.

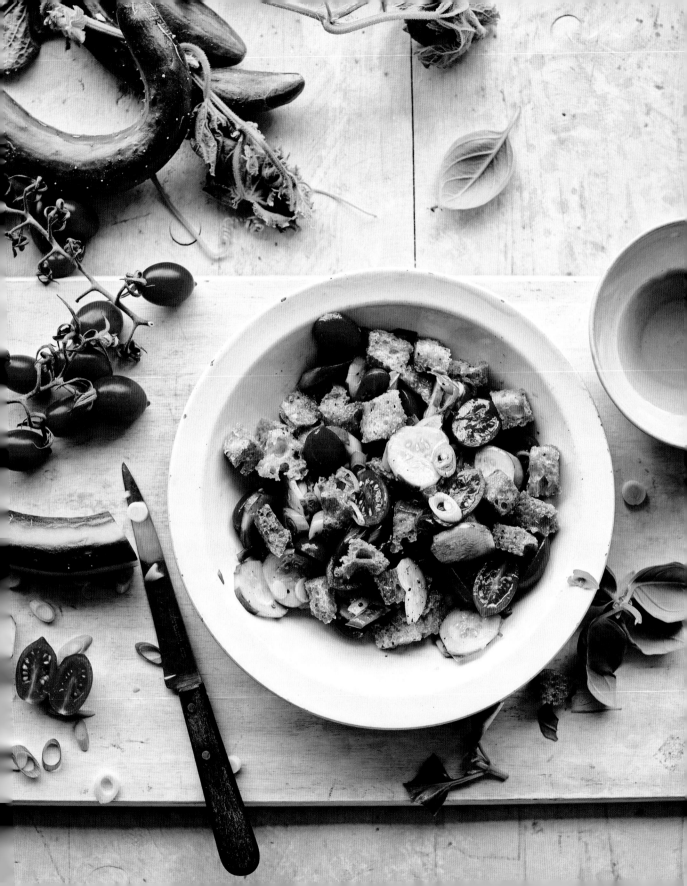

Pomodori Ripieni di Riso
Tomatoes Stuffed with Rice, Anchovies and Capers

Tomatoes lend themselves to be stuffed and the stuffings can be quite varied: pasta, sausages, shrimps and mayonnaise, scrambled eggs and herbs and more. The simplest recipe, and one of the best, is vegetables stuffed with breadcrumbs, parsley and garlic as in *Melanzane Ripiene alla Siciliana* (see page 108). This traditional rice stuffing combines the fresh flavour of the tomatoes with the comforting softness of the rice.

Serves 4

4 large ripe tomatoes

150g/5 ½oz/⅔ cup long grain rice

1 tbsp small capers, rinsed

8 anchovy fillets, drained

2 garlic cloves

25g/1oz/1 cup flat leaf parsley

4 tbsp extra virgin olive oil

Sea salt and freshly ground black pepper

Wash and dry the tomatoes and cut them in half along their middle. Scoop out the seeds and sprinkle them with salt. Lay them upside down on a board to drain.

Cook the rice in boiling, salted water until very al dente – rice eaten cold needs to be more al dente than when eaten hot. Drain and rinse under cold running water.

Chop the anchovies, garlic and parsley together and place in a frying pan. Add the oil and cook for 1 minute while stirring the whole time. Spoon in the rice and capers and continue cooking for a further 2–3 minutes. Season with plenty of pepper and then taste and check the salt, which may already be fine due to the saltiness of the anchovies.

Dry the inside of the tomatoes with kitchen paper and put them on a serving dish or on individual plates. Fill them with the rice stuffing and leave them until the rice is cold – which will take about 2 hours. Do not refrigerate them – they are best served at room temperature.

Porro
Leek

My suppers during the cold months would be much poorer without leeks, a very versatile vegetable. The part of the leek which is usually used is the white bulb; however, the pale green leaves inside the dark, tougher, outer ones are excellent, too. You can use the outer leaves for stock.

Hardly known in southern Italy, leeks are popular in the north where they grow. Try to buy thin leeks; the fatter ones sometimes have a hard core. They are usually cooked, although, more recently, small, young leeks are sometimes sliced very finely and added raw to a salad. They are excellent added to beetroot. To do this, first soak the sliced leeks in salted water for about 1 hour to get rid of some of their oniony flavour.

Like Nero, the emperor, I love them and eat them cooked in different ways, including soup. I sauté the white bulb cut into 5mm/¼in strips, in plenty of butter, which I far prefer to oil in this dish; or I poach it whole, cut it in half and dress it with oil, lemon juice, salt and a generous grinding of pepper. I make frittata with it or a very good pasta sauce to which I add a pinch – or two or even three – of curry powder, a recipe which has been in my repertoire ever since I first had it in Piedmont over 40 years ago. Curry in Italy? And in a pasta sauce? Yes, and it works very well.

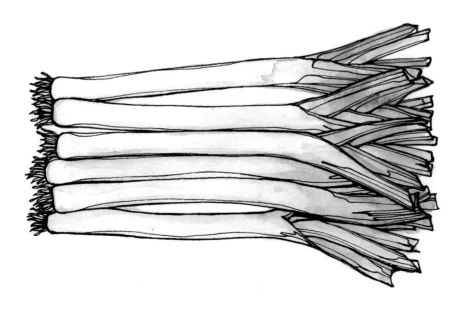

Tortino di Porri e Riso
Leek and Rice Bake

I love this dish, which I also make with courgettes. It started off as a pie encased in filo pastry; but then one day I didn't have any filo pastry in the freezer and I made it without, and it is just as good, although different. I like to serve this *tortino* surrounded, or covered, with *Pomodorini Arrostiti* or Roasted Cherry Tomatoes (see page 137).

For this dish you need only the white part of the leeks and the inside pale green leaves (keep the green foliage for a soup).

Serves 4

400g/14oz leeks, trimmed and cut into 5mm/¼in rounds

85g/3oz/½ cup arborio rice

2 eggs

100ml/3½fl oz/scant ½ cup extra virgin olive oil

4 tbsp freshly grated Parmesan

Sea salt and freshly ground black pepper

3 tbsp dried breadcrumbs

Put the leeks in a sink of cold water. Wash thoroughly, removing any earth, drain and put in a bowl. Add the rice.

Lightly beat the eggs and add to the bowl together with half the oil, 3 tbsp of the Parmesan and salt and pepper. Mix well – hands are the best tool for the job. Leave the mixture to rest for about 1 hour: the rice and the leeks will absorb some of the liquid and soften up.

Heat the oven to 160°C Fan/180°C/350°F/Gas Mark 4.

Grease an oven dish with some of the remaining oil and spoon in the mixture. Mix together the remaining Parmesan and the breadcrumbs and sprinkle over the top. Drizzle with the remaining oil and bake for 45–50 minutes. Taste by inserting the point of a knife into the middle and dig out a few grains of rice. They should be tender. Remove the dish from the oven and leave to rest for a few minutes before serving.

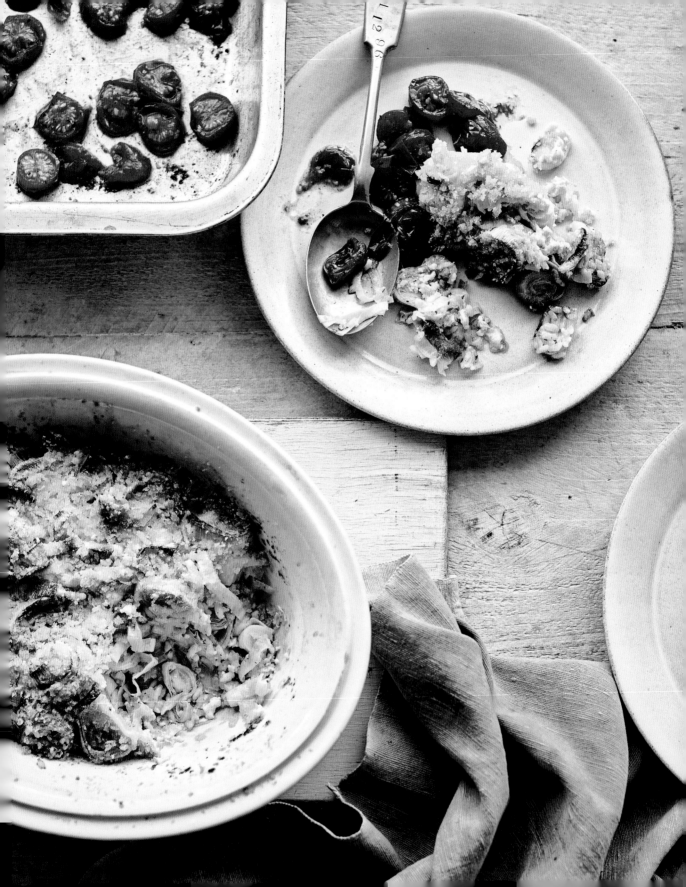

Porri alla Panna
Leeks Baked with Cream and Cheese

This winter dish from Lombardy is delicious as it is, but if you want to make it more filling cover the bottom of the oven dish with a few slices of ham, as I sometimes do.

Serves 4

500g/1lb 2oz leeks

100ml/3½fl oz/scant ½ cup vegetable stock made from bouillon powder

25g/1oz/1½ tbsp unsalted butter, cut into small pieces

Sea salt and freshly ground black pepper

100g/3½oz Gruyère

6 tbsp crème fraîche

4 tbsp freshly grated Parmesan

Heat the oven to 180°C Fan/200°C/400°F/Gas Mark 6.

Trim the leeks by discarding the outer leaves and keeping the white leaves and the pale green inner ones. Cut them in pieces about 15cm/6in long and wash very well, trying to keep the leaves together as much as you can.

Take an ovenproof dish that you can put on the stove – the sort that has a removable handle is ideal – and place the leeks side by side in it in two layers. Pour in the vegetable stock and add the butter and salt and pepper to taste. Cover the pan and cook over a gentle heat for about 10 minutes until the leeks are soft. If there is more than a thin layer of liquid at the bottom of the pan when the leeks are ready, remove the leeks from the pan and set on one side while you reduce the liquid.

Return the leeks to the pan, shave the Gruyère over the leeks and spoon the crème fraîche over. Sprinkle with the Parmesan and place the dish in the oven for about 10 minutes, until a golden crust appears on top. Remove from the oven and leave to rest for 3–4 minutes before serving.

Porri in Salsa Piccante
Leeks in a Vinaigrette Sauce

This recipe has been in my repertoire for the last 30 years or so. As with quite a few of my best recipes, I owe it to my friend Myriam, an Italian and a very good cook, who is very generous with her recipes. The vinegary sauce works very well with the sweetness of the leeks. If you haven't any stock to hand, make it with a bouillon.

Serves 4

8 medium-sized leeks

500ml/fl oz/cups beef stock

4 tbsp extra virgin olive oil

2 tbsp balsamic vinegar

Juice of ½ unwaxed lemon

1 tsp Dijon mustard

*Sea salt and freshly ground black
    pepper*

2 eggs

*6 rashers back bacon, cut into small
    strips*

1 tbsp small capers, rinsed

Heat the oven to 160°C Fan/180°C/350°F/Gas Mark 4.

Trim and thoroughly wash the leeks, leaving some of the best green tops attached. Cut each in half lengthwise. Place them in an ovenproof dish in which they will fit in no more than two layers.

Bring the stock to the boil, pour it over the leeks and place the dish in the oven. Bake the leeks for about 15–20 minutes or until tender when pierced them with the point of a small knife. Lift the leeks out and place them to dry on kitchen paper. Keep the stock for a soup – it is very good.

To make the vinaigrette, put the oil, vinegar, lemon juice, mustard and salt and pepper in a bowl and mix well. Taste and adjust the seasoning, adding a little more lemon juice to your liking.

Bring a saucepan of water to the boil and add the eggs. Boil for 4 minutes. Put the pan under cold water and then peel the the eggs.

Put a small frying pan on the heat, add the bacon and fry until the bacon is crisp. Lift it out of the pan with a slotted spoon and place it on kitchen paper to drain.

Spread one spoonful of the vinaigrette in a serving dish, lay the leeks on top (cut side up) and then spoon the rest of the vinaigrette on top.

Cut the eggs into small pieces and scatter over the top, together with the capers and bacon.

These leeks are good eaten at room temperature with plenty of crusty bread to mop up the juices.

Puntarelle
Puntarelle

One of the foods I miss most here in Dorset is *puntarelle*, or *catalogna* as my mother called them and as they are called in northern Italy. They are a variety of chicory with long, green leaves and are in season from November until about February. With luck you can find them in food markets in London and other big cities, but Dorset, the most English of all English counties, is certainly not fertile ground for them.

Preparing them is quite a laborious job. First pull away the dark outside leaves and any other dark green leaves around some of the stalks. Then cut off the base of each stalk and cut the white stalks vertically in half and then into strips, about 3cm/1¼in wide. Now fill a basin of cold water, add some ice cubes and plunge the *puntarelle* into the water. Leave for 30 minutes or longer until the *puntarelle* have curled up as little white ribbons.

In Rome, where they are very popular, greengrocers sell ready prepared *puntarelle* swimming in barrels of water and ready to be dressed, which is a great help to the home cook.

Puntarelle alla Romana
Puntarelle Salad

Serves 4

1 head puntarelle
1 garlic clove
4 anchovy fillets, drained
2 tsp lemon juice
4 tbsp extra virgin olive oil
Freshly ground black pepper

Prepare the *puntarelle* as described above and, after their icy bath, drain and dry them very well with kitchen paper. Put them in a bowl.

Remove the germ from the garlic clove, put the garlic in a mortar and pound it to a paste with a pestle. Add the anchovies and lemon juice and pound again while adding the oil. You can make the dressing in the small bowl of a food processor rather than a mortar and pestle, if you prefer. Because of the anchovies, you should not need to add any salt. If you want, you can add some pepper, although this is not a typical Roman addition.

Spoon the dressing over the salad, toss well and serve immediately.

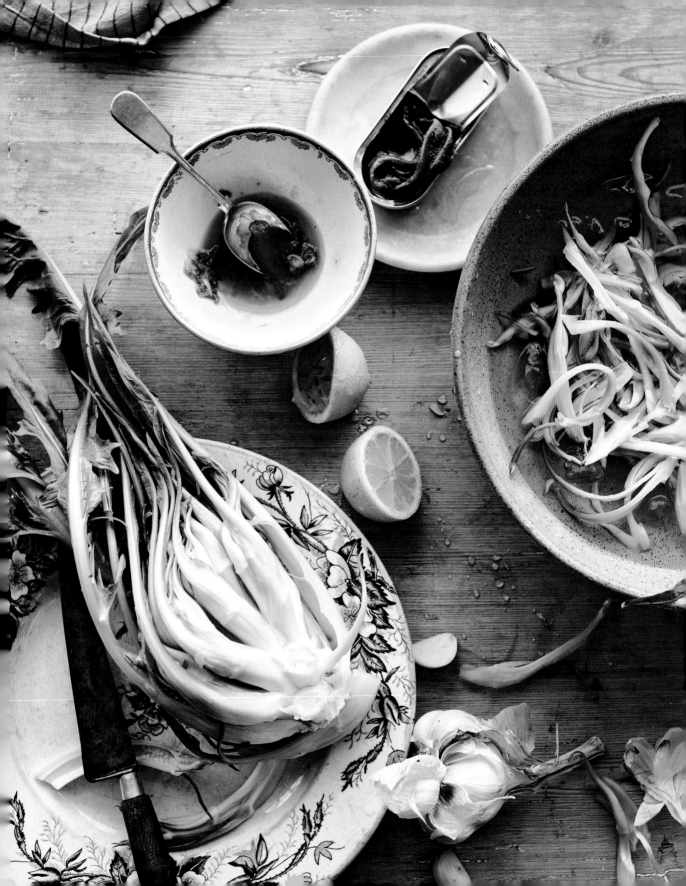

Radicchio
Radicchio

Radicchio is the generic name for the red varieties of chicory that are cultivated by a special method of forcing and blanching. In the last ten years radicchio has become a popular addition to salads. Not only does it give the bowl of salad an attractive appearance, it also gives it a crunchy, bitter flavour that makes the salad far more appetizing.

There are three main varieties of radicchio: Chioggia, Castelfranco and Treviso. The radicchio di Chioggia is the common radicchio we see everywhere. It is available all year round and is best in salads A tight red ball with a slightly bitter flavour, it gives any salad a punch and its lovely reddish hue makes the salad far more visually attractive. The Castelfranco looks like a large red and ivory variegated rose; it is excellent roasted or grilled, as is the Treviso variety with its elongated leaves and possibly the most flavourful of the three. One of the best lunches I ever had was indeed in Treviso, a town which has a reputation for good food; it started with a perfectly cooked *risotto al radicchio*, followed by a *pollo in tecia* (chicken cooked at length in an earthenware pot) and finished with one of the best tiramisùs ever – Treviso is the birthplace of this ubiquitous pudding.

You can make a good salad with finely cut radicchio mixed with pieces of Gorgonzola and a scattering of walnuts on top and dressed with lemon juice and olive oil.

Insalata di Radicchio, Scarola e Arancia
Red Radicchio, Endive and Orange Salad

Oranges go very well in a salad, but you need to buy the least sweet variety possible. Blood oranges work well but, alas, have a very short season. If your oranges are very sweet, add more lemon juice.

Serves 4

200g/7oz red radicchio

200g/7oz curly endive (friseé)

1 fennel bulb

1 orange

3 tbsp extra virgin olive oil

1 tsp Dijon mustard

Lemon juice to taste

Sea salt and freshly ground black pepper

Wash, drain and dry the radicchio and endive and cut into strips. Remove the stalk and any brown or bruised part of the outside of the fennel, but reserve a few fronds. Cut it vertically into thin segments. Wash, drain and dry them. Peel the orange to the quick – which means removing the skin and also all the pith – and cut into slices.

Now make the dressing. Take a large salad bowl and pour in the olive oil. Mix in the mustard, using a fork to incorporate, add the lemon juice and season with salt and some pepper if you want, although the mustard gives the dish enough heat. Taste and adjust the dressing as you prefer.

Add the salad and the fennel to the bowl, toss well and then place the orange slices across the top. Sprinkle with the fennel fronds.

Radicchio Rosso e Cicoria alla Trevisana
Grilled Radicchio and Chicory

The *radicchio rosso* or red radicchio used in Veneto for this dish is the long radicchio of Treviso, which can be bought during the autumn in many specialist greengrocers. It has a deeper, and yet more delicate, bitter flavour than the round Rosa di Chioggia, the variety of radicchio rosso widely available all the year round.

For a vegetarian dish, omit the anchovy fillets and increase the capers to 2 tbsp.

Serves 6

2 radicchio rosso bunches

4 chicory

6 tbsp extra virgin olive oil

Sea salt and freshly ground black
   pepper

1 garlic clove, chopped

8 anchovy fillets, drained and chopped

1 tbsp capers, rinsed

2 tbsp balsamic vinegar

Heat the grill/broiler.

Wash and dry the salad. Cut the red radicchio in quarters and the chicory in half, both lengthwise.

Place the radicchio and chicory cut side up in a deep baking dish and spoon about 4 tbsp of the oil over. Season with salt and pepper and cook under the hot grill for about 8 minutes, taking care to turn the heat down if the vegetables are becoming burnt. Turn the pieces over halfway during the grilling. They are cooked when the core can easily be pierced by the point of a knife. Lay the grilled pieces on a serving dish.

Heat the remaining oil in a small frying pan and add the garlic, anchovy fillets and capers. Sauté gently for a minute or two and then add the balsamic vinegar and cook for a further minute. Season with salt and a generous grinding of pepper and pour on top of the radicchio and chicory.

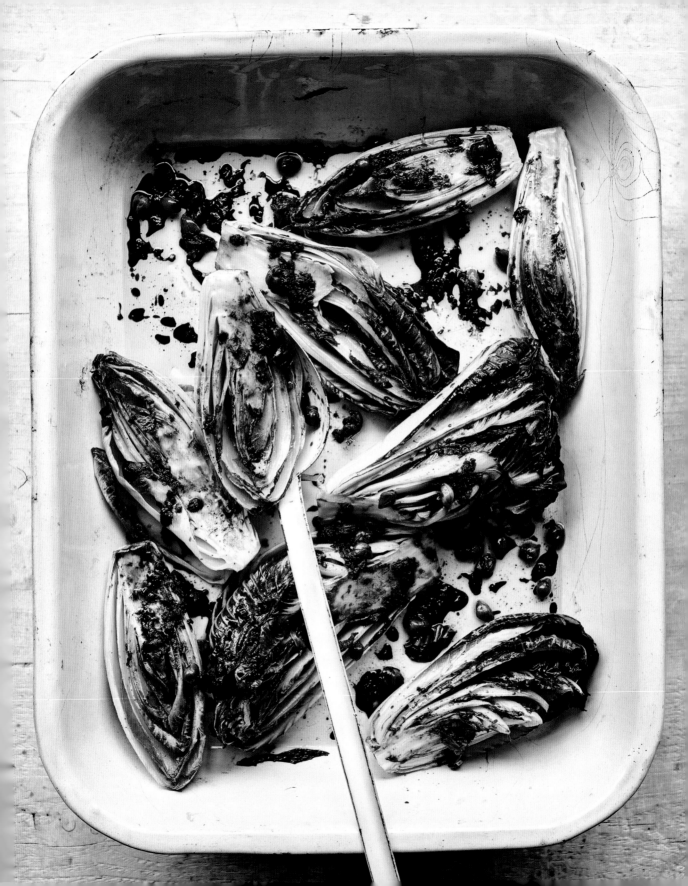

Rapa
Turnip

All in all, I think I could live quite happily without ever eating turnips again. I still remember the *riso e rape* – rice and turnip soup – sitting in front of a young me; I slowly pushed it round and round the bowl with the spoon hoping that it might disappear; but it didn't and I had to eat it, as we children had to do with any food put in front of us. But you might love turnips so I am including a recipe I hope you will like.

Turnips were very popular in Roman times. In Apicius' book there are as many recipes for them as there are for carrots, with which they are also mixed, as in a recipe in which both vegetables are stewed in wine and sweetened with honey – an excellent idea. Bartolomeo Platina, in his famous book *De honesta voluptate* written during the second half of the 15th century, mentions the beneficial qualities of turnips, including increasing the sperm count. He also writes that Columella, the Roman agriculturalist, warns that 'we must be careful when we gather turnips that they do not harbour some little poisonous worms, which would die if a menstruating woman would walk three times around the vegetable garden with her hair loose and without shoes'. What a lot of rubbish from such a great man.

Turnips used to be a very popular vegetable in northern Italy especially in the regions which were part of the Austro-Hungarian Empire until the end of the First World War – Trentino-Alto Adige and Friuli-Venezia Giulia. Now they seem to have lost some of their prestige. This is a pity because when young and fresh they are excellent – for young I mean they should be hard to the touch, with a tight skin and a fresh-looking sprouting stalk. In Italy they are usually baked in layers with cheese and often also served with a béchamel sauce. They are also good sautéed in plenty of butter flavoured with onion.

Rapa alla Trentina
Glazed Turnips

In Milan before the Second World War when I was a child we had a cook from Friuli, Maria. I loved her and spent hours in the kitchen with her: watching, helping, listening to and bothering her. Her potato gnocchi are still the best gnocchi I have ever eaten, as were her *polpette* meat rissoles, into which, during the truffle season, she used to stick a tiny bit of white truffle – food for the poor (the rissoles) elevated to food for princes.

This is the recipe for Maria's turnips, a vegetable which, she used to say, saved her and her siblings from starvation during the winter months. I expect quite a few of you, my readers, have seen the film 'L'Albero degli Zoccoli', 'The Tree of the Clogs', which is set in Lombardy before the First World War. In Friuli the life of the peasants was like that up to the end of the Second World War. Like all her sisters and friends, Maria, who was born in 1910, was sent into domestic service when she was 13, as a tweenie. She learned her metier from the cook of the house, who was apparently very good and very kind to her and Maria blossomed in her career. She came to us when she was 20, already well qualified to be a cook, but more a family cook, as my mother required, rather than a cook for a grand household, which ours was certainly not.

Maria or no Maria, I did not like turnips then but I like them cooked as in this recipe, which emphasizes their distinctive flavour, making it more delicate and subtle.

Serves 4

600g/1lb 5oz small, young turnips
2 tsp white sugar
30g/1oz/2 tbsp unsalted butter,
  cut into small pieces
A grating of nutmeg
½ tsp ground cinnamon
Sea salt

Wash the turnips, cut off the stalks and the dangling root and then cut them into half or quarters, depending on their size. Cut each piece into 1cm/½in slices and put into a sauté pan. Cover with warm water to come level with the layer of turnips.

Add the sugar and the butter. Cover the pan and bring to the boil. Remove the lid and cook at a very low simmer for about 20–30 minutes until the turnips are tender and there is no more liquid at the bottom of the pan. Keep an eye on them; they should not catch at the bottom. If they are not yet soft and there is no liquid in the pan, add some boiling water.

About halfway through the cooking, add the spices and salt to taste. In Friuli no pepper is added, but you can add it if you like. Taste the dish before you serve to check the salt.

Rapanello
Radish

In a vegetable beauty contest, radishes would surely win – and they are also good to eat. They are lovely thinly sliced and added to a green salad or mixed with sliced cucumber. Radishes are also invaluable for decorating a dish and they are even prettier with their leaves left on. They are often used in a *Bagna Caôda* (see page 30) and always as part of the display of vegetables in the Roman *pinzimonio*. I love them also served with sliced mozzarella and a balsamic vinegar dressing.

When they are fresh, you can use the green tops for a pasta sauce – the best pasta for this sauce is wholewheat spaghetti. Discard the thick stalks and blanch the leaves for 1 minute. Drain thoroughly and chop the leaves. Sauté them in some olive oil flavoured with garlic, chilli and anchovy fillets.

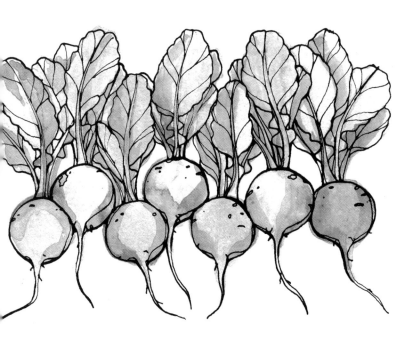

Insalata di Rapanelli e Cetrioli
Radish and Cucumber Salad

This salad is as pretty to look at as it is good to eat. Very often it has come to my rescue when, short of any vegetables for a salad, I have found half a cucumber and a few radishes lying at the bottom of the refrigerator salad drawer.

Buy small cucumbers, as they have more flavour. I like to use fresh mint with cucumber, but you might prefer some other herb, like chives or parsley, which go equally well.

Serves 4

4 small or 1 large cucumber

16–18 radishes

3 tbsp extra virgin olive oil

1 tbsp balsamic vinegar

2 tsp Dijon mustard

Sea salt

About 12 mint leaves, torn

Wash and dry the cucumber and peel it in strips – this is more for looks than for anything else. Slice it very thinly and put the slices in a salad bowl.

Cut off the ends of the radishes and wash and dry them. Slice thinly and add to the salad bowl.

In a small bowl, beat together the oil and vinegar. Beat in the mustard and 2–3 pinches of salt. Beat well and then pour the dressing over the salad. Taste and check the salt and then scatter the mint over the top.

Scorzonera
Black Salsify

I always think it sad that this delicious root is not better known. It is easy to grow and makes a welcome change from the ubiquitous cabbage during the winter months when most of the vegetables on sale are not locally grown. Black salsify has a delectable flavour slightly reminiscent of truffle. Peeled and washed, it is usually boiled for about 30 minutes, cut into rounds and sautéed in butter and/or oil flavoured with onion and/or garlic. It can also be served in a warm winter salad with beetroot and boiled shallots. I also like it roasted, well coated in olive oil, mixed with carrots and young turnips. But the best method is to deep fry it. The root, previously cooked but still slightly underdone, is coated in flour, egg and breadcrumbs and fried in oil. You break through the hot, crispy crust to reach a soft, buttery mash exploding in your mouth.

Scorzonera alla Ligure
Black Salsify with Egg and Lemon

Serves 3–4

1 unwaxed lemon, cut in half

500g/1lb 2oz black salsify

4 tbsp olive oil

1 onion, finely chopped

2 tbsp chopped flat leaf parsley

Sea salt

1 tbsp flour

250ml/9fl oz/³⁄4 cup vegetable stock

2 egg yolks

Freshly ground black pepper

The final addition of the lemony egg sauce intensifies the earthy asparagus-truffle flavour of the *scorzonera*.

Prepare a bowl full of cold water and add half the lemon. To clean the salsify, pare away the black outside layer of the roots, cut the roots into 5cm/2in pieces and cut each piece in half or, if the root is thicker than your small finger, into quarters. As soon as each piece is cut, add to the bowl of acidulated water.

Add the oil, onion, parsley and a pinch or two of salt to a sauté pan and gently cook for 5 minutes, stirring frequently. Drain the salsify, add to the *soffritto* and sauté for some 5 minutes, stirring frequently to coat the pieces. Stir in the flour and cook for a further minute, stirring the whole time. Now add about 100ml/3½fl oz/⅓ cup of the stock, mix well and cover the pan. Cook over a very low heat for about 45–50 minutes, until the roots are tender. Keep an eye and add some more stock if needed.

Gently beat the egg yolks together, add the juice of the remaining lemon half and a grinding of pepper. When the salsify is tender, remove the pan from the heat and mix in the egg and lemon mixture. The yolks will cook just a little but still be pretty runny. Taste and check the seasoning.

Sedano
Celery

This is a very basic ingredient in Italian cooking, so much so that in the old days – mine – greengrocers used to give their customers a small bag containing one stick of celery, a few sprigs of parsley, two or three bay leaves and sometimes a few garlic cloves, which were called *gli odori* or 'the smells'. They were considered necessary in any kitchen as the basis of most dishes. And that celery certainly is and has been so since Roman times. In Ancient Rome and Athens, celery was also used as a decoration and for making crowns to put on the heads of athletes and poets, just like bay leaves were.

There are two varieties of celery in Italy, the green and the white. The green has green stalks and a stronger flavour and is used for making the *soffritto* – the beaten mixture which is the point of departure of many dishes. White celery has a more delicate flavour and is used thinly sliced in salads. The habit of eating celery and cheese together does not exist in Italy and I feel the Italians are missing something here, because the marriage of a good tender celery stalk with some good blue cheese is perfection.

The oddest use of celery I ever came across was in Puglia. I was in Altamura – a town famous for its *duomo* and its bread – with the artist Val Archer when we were researching our book *The painter, the cook and the art of Cucina*. We were having dinner in a modest trattoria behind the *duomo*. In the middle of the table there was a jug of red wine with 2–3 celery stalks stuck into it. 'Oh', I said to the proprietor, 'is that for giving the wine a special celery flavour?' 'No, signora, it is because the wine is not good and I thought it might taste a bit better with this treatment.'

Buy celery which has fresh green leaves and a white-looking stalk where it is cut at the bottom. Wash well as there is often some earth stuck in the hollows, and then remove the outer strings, which can be done using a small knife or a potato peeler. This is especially necessary for the coarse, outer stalks.

Insalata di Sedano, Gorgonzola e Noci
Celery, Gorgonzola and Walnut Salad

For this salad you need Gorgonzola piccante, which is dry and strong, not Dolcelatte. I have also used Dorset Blue Vinney, my local blue cheese, and mild Stilton.

A good brand of ready made mayonnaise works fine here.

Serves 2

3 celery stalks

50g/1¾oz Gorgonzola, cut into
    2cm/¾in cubes

25g/1oz walnut kernels

2 tbsp lemon juice

1 dsp mayonnaise

1 tsp Dijon mustard

1 dsp wine vinegar

2 tbsp extra virgin olive oil

Sea salt and freshly ground black
    pepper

Using a potato peeler, remove the strings from the celery stalks and wash and dry them. Cut the bottom wide part of the sticks in half and then cut the sticks in 2cm/¾in pieces. Put them in a bowl. Add the cubes of Gorgonzola to the bowl.

Chop the walnuts until they are as small as rice grains and add to the bowl. Add the lemon juice, season with salt and mix.

For the dressing, put the mayonnaise and mustard into a small bowl and mix in the vinegar and oil. Beat well and then mix into the salad. Add some pepper and toss the whole thing together very thoroughly. Taste and check the salt. If you have time, allow the salad to rest for some 20–30 minutes before serving.

Zuppa di Sedano
Celery Soup

This soup comes from Calabria, the region consisting of the toe of the Italian boot. Calabria is still probably the poorest region of Italy after its neighbour, Basilicata. What industry there is is mostly connected to agricultural produce and what there is is partly in the hands of the local mafia, the *'ndrageda*.

This is a typical soup of the region, a soup which is a meal in its own right, based on inexpensive ingredients, such as celery.

Serves 4

400g/14oz celery stalks, with leaves
if possible for garnishing
2 garlic cloves, chopped
3 tbsp olive oil
200g/7oz pork sausages
2 eggs, hard-boiled
4 slices brown bread
100g/3½oz/1½ cups mature pecorino,
grated
Freshly ground black pepper

Wash and drain the celery. Reserve the leaves for garnishing. Strip the strings from the coarse, outer stalks by breaking off a small piece of string and pulling it down or using a potato peeler. Cut the stalks into 2cm/¾in pieces and put them in a saucepan together with the garlic. Add 1.2 litres/ 2 pints/5 cups of water, the oil and 2 pinches of salt. Bring to the boil.

Cut the sausages into 2cm/¾in pieces, add to the saucepan and cook until the celery is tender, which will take about 30–45 minutes.

Cut the eggs in half and then into wedges.

Toast the bread and place one slice of toasted bread into each soup bowl. Ladle about one-quarter of the soup over each slice, place some egg wedges on top and cover with a sprinkling of pecorino and some freshly ground black pepper. If your celery has some leaves, wash and chop them, and sprinkle them over the soup. They liven up the soup both in look and in flavour.

Sedano di Verona
Celeriac

The name itself tells you that celeriac is a vegetable of northern Italy – Verona is a city between Milan and Venice – and it is hardly known in the south. I am sorry for the southerners because they miss the pleasure of a very delicious winter vegetable. It is also called *sedano rapa* – turnip celery – because of its resemblance to a large turnip.

The first mention of celeriac is in *The Iliad* where Homer writes that Achilles fed his horse with it to cure him from its illness – he didn't tell us if it was successful. In fact, celeriac does not have many medicinal properties, unlike other vegetables, although it is a very good diuretic.

Celeriac is in season from September throughout the winter. It can be eaten in salads – shredded, often with carrots, and dressed with olive oil, vinegar, mustard and mashed anchovy fillets, similar to the French *rémoulade* – or it can be baked in layers with cheese and butter or with béchamel sauce. Many chefs are now making risotto with celeriac rather than celery because it is sweeter.

The best celeriac should weigh around 600g/1lb 5oz, be firm to the touch and with few dangling roots.

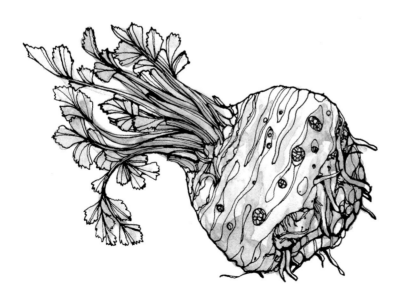

Sedano di Verona e Melanzane in Sughetto
Celeriac and Aubergine Braised in Tomato Sauce

This recipe combines two vegetables which, on paper, sound like they should never be brought together but it is an extraordinarily good combination of flavours and I hope you will have the courage to try it. Serve the dish as an accompaniment to roast meat or chicken or just by itself.

Serves 4

1 small celeriac, about 750g/1lb 10oz

1 aubergine (eggplant), about 250–300g/9–10½oz

3 tbsp olive oil

25g/1oz/2 tbsp unsalted butter

25g/1oz/1 cup flat leaf parsley, chopped

1 garlic clove, chopped

1 tbsp tomato purée (paste)

About 100ml/3½fl oz/scant ½ cup vegetable stock

Sea salt and freshly ground black pepper

Heat the oven to 160°C Fan/180°C/350°F/Gas Mark 4.

Peel the celeriac and cut it into 2cm/¾in cubes. Wash the aubergine and cut it into similar sized cubes. Put them both in a bowl and pour 1 tbsp olive oil over. Mix together with your hands to coat the cubes all over.

Heat the remaining oil and the butter in a pan which you can put later in the oven. Add the parsley and garlic, gently cook for a minute until the garlic begins to turn golden and then add the vegetable cubes. Mix well, turning the vegetables over and over and cook gently for 3–4 minutes. Add the tomato purée and continue cooking for a further 2–3 minutes. Pour in about half the stock, mix well, season with salt and pepper and bring to the boil.

Cover the pan and put it in the oven. Cook until the vegetables are done, which will take about 30–40 minutes. If necessary, add a little more stock. The vegetables should cook in a little liquid, but they should be fairly dry when they are ready. Serve hot.

Sedano di Verona e Spinaci al Gratin
Celeriac and Spinach Bake

This dish is typical of the cuisine of northern Italy in its combination of vegetables and béchamel baked in the oven. I like to cook the celeriac in meat stock for a stronger flavour, but I have often cooked it in vegetable stock or even in water. If you haven't got any fresh stock, you can always use bouillon.

Béchamel sauce is as common in northern Italy as it is in France. The great cookery writer Marcella Hazan wrote: 'Long before France christened Béchamel, a sauce of flour and milk cooked in butter was a part of the cooking of Romagna. It is essential to many of its pasta and vegetables, and such an unquestionably native dish as lasagne could not exist without it.'

Serves 4
500g/1lb 2oz celeriac
1 litre/1 ¾ pints/4 cups stock
300g/10½oz cooked or frozen spinach
*   leaves, thawed*
15g/½oz/1 tbsp unsalted butter
2 tbsp freshly grated Parmesan
2 tbsp dried white breadcrumbs

For the béchamel sauce
500ml/18fl oz/2 cups full-fat (whole)
*   milk*
50g/1¾oz/4 tbsp unsalted butter
50g/1¾oz flour
A grating of nutmeg
Sea salt

Peel the celeriac and cut into large pieces. Put the pieces in a saucepan, cover with the stock and bring to the boil. Cook for 30 minutes until tender and then drain.

Whether cooked and cooled or frozen and thawed, using your hands, squeeze out all the liquid from the spinach and cut into strips.

Heat the oven to 170°C Fan/190°C/375°F/Gas Mark 5.

To make the béchamel sauce put the milk in a tall saucepan and bring to the simmer. I use a tall one to boil milk so that it takes longer to overflow and inundate the hob – which is a bore to clean. Melt the butter in a heavy-based pan and when the foam begins to subside, mix in the flour and beat fast to incorporate. Then slowly add the milk, stirring the whole time. Take the pan off the heat every now and then to give a good stir and then start again. When all the milk has been added, add some salt to taste and cook the sauce for 4–5 minutes on a very low simmer. This is long enough to cook the flour. Add a grating of nutmeg and mix.

Grease a medium to large ovenproof dish with a little of the butter. Cut the celeriac in 5mm/¼in slices and cover the bottom of the dish with a layer of slices. Spread a little of the béchamel sauce over the celeriac and then spread the spinach on top. Dribble a little more of the béchamel over the spinach and then cover with the remaining slices of celeriac. Spread the remaining béchamel across the top.

Mix together the Parmesan and breadcrumbs and sprinkle the mixture over the dish. Dot with the remaining butter and bake for 20 minutes or until a golden crust has formed on the top. Remove from the oven and leave to rest for 2–3 minutes before serving.

Spinaci
Spinach

My diet would be very deprived without spinach. I love it for its flavour as well as for its versatility – it is good simply steamed and blessed with a few drops of good olive oil, sautéed in butter and oil, mashed and made into croquettes, added to egg pasta, made into gnocchi or used in soups. I love spinach in a risotto, too.

Spinach was brought to Sicily by the Arabs, via Spain, around 800AD. The first mention of it appears in the 14th century by Martino da Como. By the time of the Renaissance spinach was quite common in Italy and it is said that it was brought to France by Caterina de' Medici when she married Henry II in 1530. The Florentine Caterina, rightly or wrongly, is accredited with introducing many products and dishes to the French – many dishes containing spinach are called *à la florentine*.

In North America and Britain spinach became very popular thanks also to the strip cartoon Popeye the sailor, created by the American Elzie Crisler Segar. Popeye was invincible because of the amount of spinach he ate. Popeye or not, spinach is an extremely nutritious and healthy food.

There are several varieties of spinach – I find the best is the bunch variety. It comes with its roots which you need to discard and then wash the bunch very thoroughly. Beet spinach, the most popular, is often available in August and September and is worth looking out for –remove the coarser stalks before using. Nowadays a lot of spinach comes sold in plastic bags – small leaves with not much flavour, all clean and ready for a quick wash. No labour is more important than flavour.

The quantity of spinach you need to buy depends on the variety. Beet spinach has very little waste whereas small spinach leaves sold in packets has no waste at all, while bunch spinach, which is by far the best variety, has considerable waste, so you must buy something like a third more. In several recipes I give the quantity of the spinach already cooked, because its weight when raw can vary dramatically according to the type of spinach being used.

Sformato di Spinaci
Spinach Mould

A *sformato* is a very old kind of Italian vegetable dish similar to a soufflé yet much easier to make, because there is no risk of having a *sformato tombé*, as sometimes happens with a soufflé. If you want to make a more complete one-dish course, serve it with the *Funghi Trifolati* or Sautéed Mushrooms (see page 93) in autumn and winter and with the *Pomodorini Arrostiti* or Roasted Cherry Tomatoes (see page 137) in spring and summer.

Use a ring mould if you have one, and fill the hole in the middle of the turned-out mould with the accompanying sauce; or you can bake it in a soufflé dish and serve it unmoulded.

Serves 6–8

50g/1¾oz/4 tbsp unsalted butter

1 banana shallot, very finely chopped

750g/1lb 10oz cooked or frozen spinach, thawed

3 eggs

200ml/7fl oz/generous ¾ cup double (heavy) cream

100g/3½oz/1½ cups Parmesan, freshly grated

A grating of nutmeg

Grated rind of ½ unwaxed lemon

Sea salt and freshly ground black pepper

2 tbsp dried breadcrumbs

Heat the oven to 170°C Fan/190°C/375°F/Gas Mark 5.

Set aside a small knob of butter and heat the remainder in a large sauté pan. When the butter begins to turn gold, add the shallot and gently sauté for 5 minutes. Keep an eye on it and don't let the shallot become too coloured.

Squeeze the water out of the spinach, using your hands, and when as dry as you can make it, add it to the pan. Mix thoroughly so the spinach can absorb the butter evenly. Now blend the spinach in a food processor or chop it by hand. If you do it in the food processor you must be careful not to whizz for too long. The spinach should be roughly puréed to keep some of its texture intact.

Break the eggs into a large bowl and gently beat them. Gradually add the cream and then mix in the Parmesan, a generous grating of nutmeg, the lemon rind and the seasoning. Mix gently but thoroughly. Fold in the spinach a spoonful at a time. When the spinach has been added, make sure all the ingredients are well incorporated.

With the remaining butter, grease a 1 litre/1¾ pint aluminium ring mould or soufflé dish, add the breadcrumbs and shake the mould to cover the whole surface. Spoon the spinach mixture into the mould. Place the mould in a large roasting tin and pour in enough boiling water to come two-thirds of the way up the side. Place the tin in the oven and cook for 40–45 minutes, until a skewer, a piece of dried spaghetti or a wooden stick inserted in the middle of the mould comes out clean.

Remove from the oven and leave to rest for 3–4 minutes and then gently slide a spatula around the inside edge. Now with any luck, it will be ready to come out. Place a large, round dish over the mould and turn both the mould and the dish upside down. Give a gentle shake to the mould and lift it off. Spoon some of your chosen sauce in the central hole and bring your dish triumphantly to the table with the remaining sauce in a sauceboat.

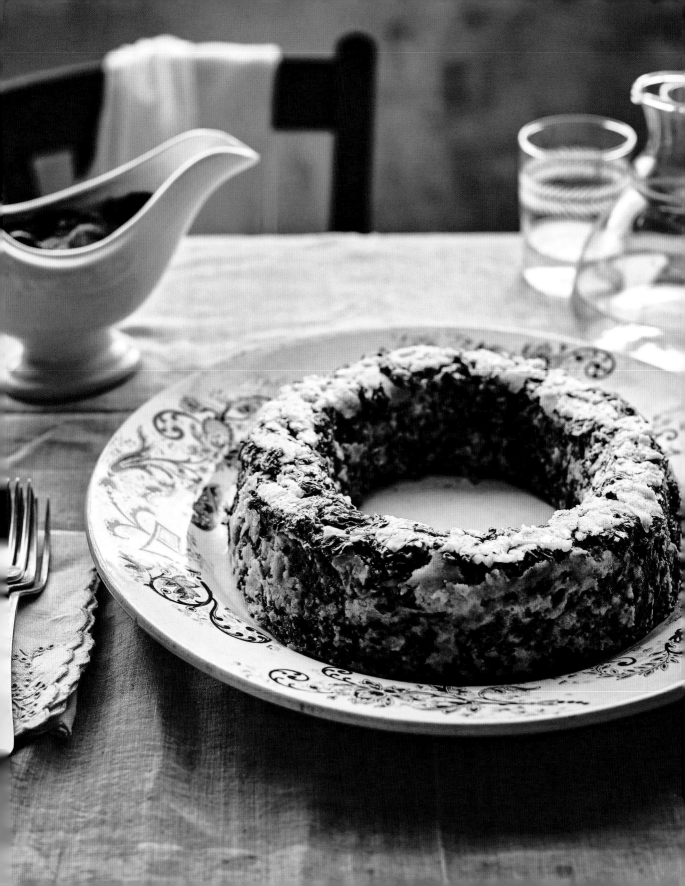

Spinaci alla Romana
Spinach with Sultanas and Pine Nuts

Making spinach *alla Romana* is the easiest and maybe the best way of using spinach. Sometimes I use anchovy fillets instead of sultanas as is done in Liguria, while at other times I finish it off the Lombard way, just with masses of butter, nutmeg and Parmesan.

The quantity of spinach needed depends on the variety. Beet spinach, the most popular, has very little waste.

Serves 4

25g/1oz sultanas

1kg/2lb 4oz fresh spinach

4 tbsp extra virgin olive oil

25g/1oz pine nuts

1 garlic clove, chopped

Sea salt and freshly ground black
   pepper

Put the sultanas in a small bowl, cover with hot water and leave to soak for some 10 minutes. Drain and dry with kitchen paper.

Wash the spinach thoroughly, discard any wilted leaves and cut off the toughest stalks. Put the spinach in a saucepan with just the water clinging to its leaves, add 1 tsp of salt and cook for 3–5 minutes, covered, until the spinach is tender. Drain into a colander and, as soon as the spinach is cool enough to handle, squeeze out the liquid using your hands. Put the ball of squeezed spinach on a chopping board and slice it.

Heat the oil in a large frying pan, add the pine nuts and garlic and sauté for 1 minute while turning the pine nuts over and over. Add the spinach and continue cooking for 5 minutes, turning it over and over in the oil. Discard the garlic. Add the dried sultanas, check the salt and season with pepper. Give the finished dish a good mix and serve.

Gnocchi Verdi
Spinach and Ricotta Gnocchi

Ricotta is a favourite ingredient in Emilia-Romagna, and these *gnocchi*, flavoured with spinach, are quite delicious. Don't worry if they are not all the same size. Incidentally, they are also called *malfatti*, meaning badly made, but the name refers only to their shape.

Serves: 4

1kg/2lb 4oz fresh spinach, or 500g/
  1lb 2oz frozen leaf spinach, thawed
2 eggs
200g/7oz ricotta cheese
200g/7oz flour
½ tsp grated nutmeg
100g/3½oz/1½ cups Parmesan,
  freshly grated
100g/3½oz/7 tbsp unsalted butter
Sea salt and freshly ground black
  pepper

Wash the spinach thoroughly, discard any wilted leaves and cut off the toughest stalks. Put the spinach in a saucepan with 1 tsp of salt and cook for about 3–5 minutes, covered. Drain into a colander and as soon as the spinach is cool enough to handle, squeeze out all the water with your hands. Chop the spinach very finely or pass it through the coarsest setting of a food mill.

In a bowl, beat the eggs together and mix in the ricotta. Beat again. Mix in the flour, spinach, nutmeg and half the Parmesan. Taste and adjust the seasoning, if necessary.

Dust your hands with flour and form the mixture into balls, the size of large marbles. Place them on a tray and chill in the refrigerator for about 30 minutes.

To cook the gnocchi, bring 4 litres/7 pints/1 gallon of salted water to the boil in a very large saucepan. Add the gnocchi, a dozen at a time. Retrieve them with a slotted spoon 3–4 minutes after the water returns to the boil, transfer them to a dish, dot with a little butter, sprinkle with a little Parmesan, and keep them warm while you continue cooking the remaining pieces.

Meanwhile, melt the remaining butter in a small saucepan. Just before serving, spoon the butter over the cooked gnocchi. Sprinkle with the remaining Parmesan and serve at once.

Rotolo di Spinaci
Spinach Roll

Usually this roll is made with homemade pasta dough but this is my mother's recipe made with potato gnocchi dough. It requires love and time but I am sure your labour and time will be amply rewarded.

Serves 4–6

650–750g/1lb 7oz–1lb 10oz floury (starchy) potatoes, scrubbed

Salt

2 tbsp olive oil

125g/4½oz/8 tbsp unsalted butter

1 small leek, cleaned, cut into thin strips and washed thoroughly

300g/10½oz frozen spinach, thawed and squeezed dry

150g/5½oz ricotta

100g/3½oz/1½ cups Parmesan, freshly grated

A grating of nutmeg

Sea salt and freshly ground black pepper

1 egg

100–150g/3½–5½oz flour

6–7 sage leaves, roughly torn

1 garlic clove, crushed

Put the potatoes in a large saucepan and cover with water. Add 1 tbsp of salt and cook them until easily pierced by the point of a knife. Drain and peel them as soon as they are cool enough to handle.

Put the oil and 25g/1oz/2 tbsp of the butter in a saucepan and, when the butter has melted, add the leek and a pinch of salt. Cover firmly and let the leek sweat for about 20–25 minutes at the lowest possible simmer.

Put the ball of spinach on a board and slice it. Add to the leek, turn the heat up to high and allow the spinach to absorb the leek liquid, while dragging it around the pan. Add the mixture to a bowl. Add the ricotta, 4 tbsp of the Parmesan, a generous grating of nutmeg and a good deal of pepper. Mix very thoroughly and then taste and check the salt.

Now go back to the potatoes. Pass the potatoes through a food mill or potato ricer straight onto the work surface. Make a well in the middle of the potato mound and break the egg into it. Gradually add enough flour to shape the mixture into a ball. It is difficult to estimate the exact quantity of the flour because it depends on the quality of the potatoes and also, the heat and humidity of your kitchen. Whatever you do, don't add all the flour at once; add it gradually and stop when the dough is firm enough to be shaped into a ball, albeit still on the sticky side, just as when making potato gnocchi. Allow the dough to cool a little.

Cut a piece of parchment paper into a rectangle of 50 x 40cm/20 x 16in and place it on the work surface. Put the dough on top of the parchment and roll it out into a rectangle about 35 x 25cm/14 x 10in. Spread the spinach filling evenly over the dough, leaving a clean edge of about 2cm/¾in all around. With the help of the parchment paper, roll the potato dough into a sausage shape, just as you would do with a Swiss roll. Press down each end and wrap the paper around the roll.

Continued overleaf

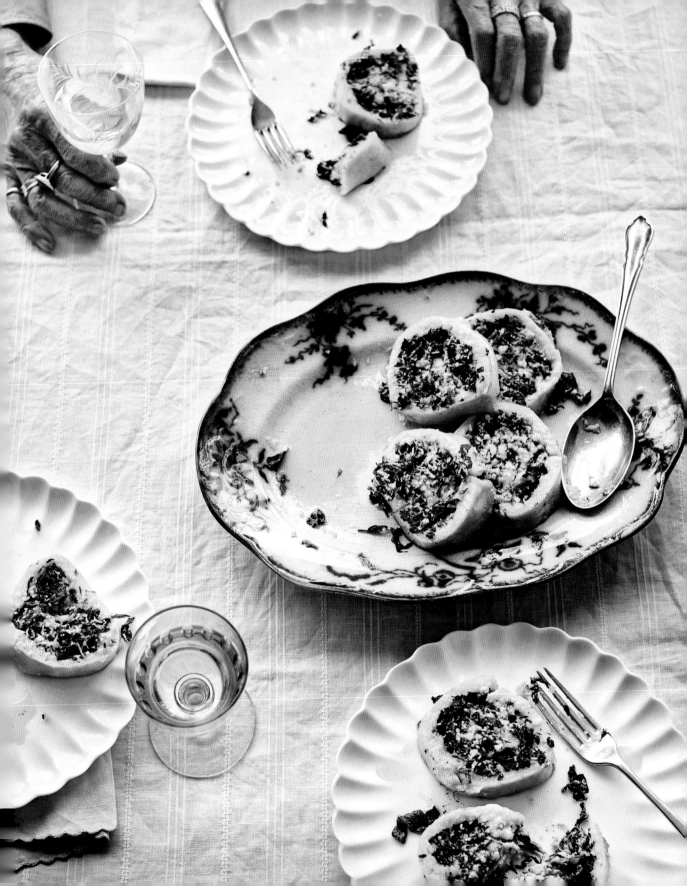

Take a large oval saucepan or a fish kettle and half fill it with water. Add 1 tbsp of salt and bring the water to the boil. Gently lower the roll into the water, which should just cover the roll. When the water is boiling again, turn the heat down to a simmer and cook for 30 minutes.

Heat the oven to 160°C Fan/180°C/350°F/Gas Mark 4.

Gently lift the roll out of the water and place on a chopping board. Leave to cool for 5 minutes before unwrapping it. It will be far easier to slice when cool. With a sharp knife, cut the roll into 2cm/¾in slices. Lay the slices in an ovenproof dish and put the dish in the oven, while you prepare the dressing, which is quick and easy.

Put the rest of the butter into a small saucepan and heat gently. Add the sage leaves and garlic to the butter. Cook gently until the foam has subsided and the butter begins to colour. Discard the garlic and pour the butter and sage leaves all over the spinach roll. Sprinkle with some of the remaining Parmesan and place the dish back in the oven for at least 15 minutes. It all depends on how cold the roll was when you put it in the oven. If it was really cold, it will take about 30 minutes to heat up again. Remove from the oven and serve, handing around the remaining cheese in a bowl.

Minestra di Spinaci
Spinach Soup

This soup is perfect in its modesty. Use bunch spinach if possible as it has more flavour than beet spinach.

Serves 4

*700g/1lb 9oz bunch spinach, roots cut
off and washed thoroughly*

50g/1¾oz/4 tbsp unsalted butter

2 garlic cloves, crushed

4 eggs

*4 tbsp freshly grated Parmesan, plus
more for the table*

A grating of nutmeg

*Sea salt and freshly ground black
pepper*

*1.2 litres/2 pints/5 cups vegetable or
chicken stock*

Put the spinach in a saucepan without adding any extra water. Cook over a high heat for 3–5 minutes until tender. Drain and when cool, squeeze out all the water using your hands. Chop the spinach finely.

Heat the butter and garlic in a frying pan and, when you smell the aroma of the garlic, add the spinach. Sauté for 5 minutes, turning the spinach over and over. Remove and discard the garlic cloves.

Gently beat the eggs in a heatproof bowl and add the Parmesan, a grating of nutmeg and salt and pepper.

Put the stock into a saucepan and bring to the boil. Pour 1 ladleful of the stock over the eggs while beating with a fork. Add the spinach to the saucepan, mix well and gently simmer for 5 minutes, while stirring occasionally. Pour in the the stock and egg mixture. Taste and check the seasoning to taste. Serve with some more Parmesan on the side for the Parmesan lovers.

Vellutata di Spinaci e Crescione
Spinach and Watercress Soup

Vellutata means 'velvety' and this soup is indeed quite velvety and delicious. It is a favourite of mine, despite it not being really Italian. The recipe was given to me by a friend, a very good English cook. I like the soup very much because the watercress here is not really cooked, just heated through, and thus it keeps its distinctive peppery flavour.

Serves 4

30g/1oz/1½ tbsp unsalted butter

2 tbsp olive oil

1 onion, chopped

1 x 150g/5½oz can cannellini beans

250ml/9fl oz/¾ cup vegetable or
   chicken stock

1 bunch watercress, washed

500g/1lb 2oz fresh spinach, roots cut
   off and washed thoroughly

Salt and freshly ground black pepper

Pouring (light) cream and crushed chilli
   (chili) flakes to serve, optional

Heat the butter and oil in a large saucepan and add the onion together with a pinch of salt. Gently sauté the onion for a few minutes, stirring frequently so that it just becomes soft and slightly coloured, not golden.

Drain and rinse the cannellini beans and add to the soup together with the stock. Bring to the boil.

Add the watercress and spinach to the saucepan and mix well. Do this a little at a time, all the while stirring so that the vegetables easily fit in the saucepan. As soon as all the vegetables are in, give the soup a good stir and turn the heat off. The watercress and the spinach should just wilt, not cook.

Use a stick blender to blend the soup for a few seconds. Add salt and pepper to taste and then ladle the soup into individual soup bowls. Serve as it is – and it is very good – or with a jug of pouring cream or, for a delicious kick, with an added pinch of crushed chilli flakes.

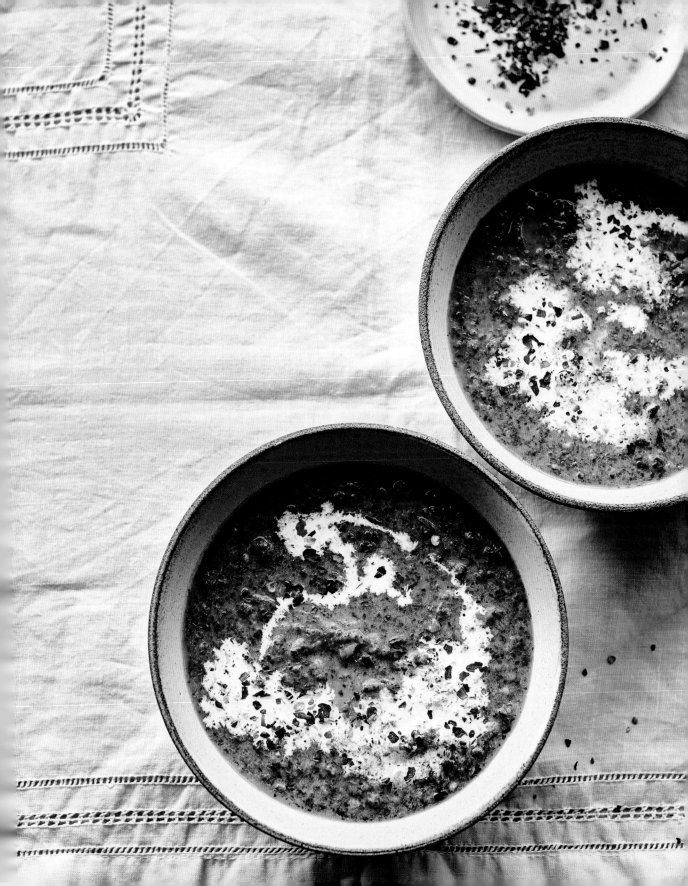

Scarpazza
Spinach Cake from Lombardy

The region of Lombardy has quite a few recipes that mix together both savoury and sweet ingredients, a combination which makes them more sophisticated.

Serves 6

50g/1¾oz 2-day old white sourdough bread

500ml/18fl oz/2 cups full fat (whole) milk

30g/1oz sultanas (golden raisins)

120g/4½oz/8 tbsp unsalted butter

50g/1¾oz flour

1kg/2lb 4oz cooked or frozen spinach, thawed

3 eggs

30g/1oz almonds, chopped

30g/1oz pine nuts, chopped

30g/1oz digestive biscuits, crumbled

½ tsp fennel seeds

½ tsp ground cinnamon

4 tbsp freshly grated Parmesan

Sea salt and freshly ground black pepper

Dried breadcrumbs for the tin

Put the bread in a small bowl, cover with the milk and set aside for 30 minutes. Then break it up with a fork and beat it to a paste.

Put the sultanas in a small bowl and cover with hot water. Leave for 20 minutes or so to plump up.

Heat the oven to 180°C Fan/200°C/400°F/Gas Mark 6.

In a medium-sized pan, melt 100g/3½oz/6 tbsp of the butter, add the flour and cook for 1 minute, stirring the whole time. Add the bread and milk mixture and continue cooking over a very low heat for 5 minutes, stirring frequently.

Meanwhile, squeeze all the liquid out of the spinach using your hands and add to the pan. Cook for a further minute or two, stirring constantly and then transfer the mixture to a bowl and leave it to cool a little.

Lightly beat the eggs together and add to the bread and spinach mixture, together with the almonds, pine nuts, digestive biscuits, fennel seeds, cinnamon and Parmesan. Drain and dry the sultanas and add to the mixture. Season with salt and pepper.

Butter a 25cm/10in springform cake tin with a little of the remaining butter and cover the buttered surface with breadcrumbs. Shake off the excess crumbs. Spoon the spinach mixture into the tin, dot with the remaining butter and cover the tin with a sheet of aluminium foil. Place the tin in the oven and cook for 20 minutes. Remove the foil and bake for a further 30–40 minutes or until a skewer, a piece of dried spaghetti or a wooden stick inserted in the middle of the cake comes out dry.

Remove from the oven and allow to cool for at least 30 minutes before you unmould it. This cake is also very good cold.

Taccola
Mangetout

This variety of the pea has been developed so that the pod can be eaten as well as the peas inside. Mangetout have a very delicate flavour, which combines better with butter than with oil. One of the best ways of preparing them is to dress cooked mangetout with melted butter and a sprinkling of grated Parmesan.

The recipe on page 176 is from Piedmont, where mangetout are well known, as they are in Lombardy, while in southern Italy they are totally unknown. Another good way of serving them is in a tomato sauce but, personally, I find that the sauce kills the flavour of the vegetable.

Mangetout should be pale green and firm. They need topping and tailing before cooking, as the string along one of their sides can be rather tough. Sometimes mangetout are served still too crunchy before they have released their full flavour, so don't cook them to a pulp, but so they still retain a 'tender bite'.

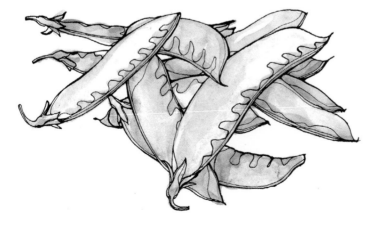

Taccole con la Panna
Mangetout with Cream and Parmesan Cheese

This delicate-flavoured vegetable needs to be treated gently with delicate ingredients, as in this recipe from Milan. Years and years ago at home in the autumn when white truffles were not just for billionaires, my mother used to grate a shaving of white truffles over the mangetout. And this is how I ate them a few years ago in a restaurant near the famous truffle town of Alba in Piedmont. Side dishes of mangetout were placed on our left and a waiter came round with a white truffle in one hand and the truffle grater in the other. He started grating while softly whispering *dieci, venti, trenta* (ten, twenty, thirty). He was counting in euros that went up rapidly according to the amount of grating. In spite of being a guest, or maybe because I was one, I stopped at *venti* and the result was certainly worth it.

Serves 4

300g/10½oz mangetout (snow peas)
250ml/9fl oz/1 cup double (heavy)
*   cream*
Sea salt
3 tbsp freshly grated Parmesan
Freshly ground black pepper

Top and tail the mangetout and wash them. Put them in a heavy-based saucepan and pour in the cream. Put the pan on a low heat and bring to the simmer. Season with salt and cover the pan.

Cook until the mangetout are tender – I like them tender which means that I cook them for about 10 minutes, but you might like them more al dente. If there is too much creamy sauce when the mangetout are ready, fish them out with a slotted spoon and boil the liquid briskly until reduced. When they are cooked to your liking, mix in the Parmesan and some pepper to taste. That's it – heavenly simplicity.

Topinambour
Jerusalem Artichoke

Like the potato and the tomato, this knobbly tuber came from Central America but, unlike those two, has never been as popular. This might well be because it is quite difficult to clean, as well as the effect it can have on some people's tummies.

Found only in northern Italy, Jerusalem artichokes have a delicate flavour, slightly sweet and reminiscent of globe artichokes. They are usually steamed or boiled before being cooked in different ways. They can also be gently braised on a bed of sliced onions. They are also good very finely sliced or shredded and eaten raw dressed with a sharp vinaigrette. Jerusalem artichokes are excellent in a risotto – lightly steam or boil them, then sauté them and add the rice. Alternatively, they can be cooked, then puréed and added to the risotto halfway through its cooking time. The cooking water is then added to the risotto.

Zuppa di Topinambour
Jerusalem Artichoke Soup

In my home in Milan, this soup was made with potato and onion and then puréed, but I like this version made with onion and rice, leaving the vegetables in small pieces. For a thicker soup you could use 1 large potato instead of the rice, added along with the onion and artichokes, then puréed once cooked in stock.

Serves 4

500g/1lb 2oz Jerusalem artichokes, scrubbed and trimmed

30g/1oz/2 tbsp unsalted butter

1 onion, thinly sliced

1.2 litres/2 pints/5 cups vegetable stock

125g/4oz/½ cup Italian rice, preferably Vialone Nano

2 tbsp chopped flat leaf parsley

Sea salt

Cut the artichokes into small cubes. Melt 20g/¾oz/1½ tbsp of the butter in a large saucepan and add the onion and artichokes and cook for some 5 minutes. The artichokes will still be slightly undercooked, but do not worry, they will finish cooking later in the stock.

Add the stock and bring to the boil. Cover and simmer gently for 20 minutes. Mix in the rice and cook until al dente. Taste and check the salt. No pepper should be added to this slightly sweet soup.

Draw the pan off the heat and stir in the rest of the butter and the parsley. Ladle the soup into individual bowls as soon as the butter has melted.

Zucca
Pumpkin and Squash

The word *zucca* covers all the varieties of this vegetable, from very large, yellow pumpkins, such as the Mantovana (see facing page) to the long Tromboncini squash from Naples. It used to be a very popular vegetable, but now it is not eaten much except in Lombardy, Veneto and Sicily. In Lombardy it is used as a stuffing for ravioli, sometimes containing also a few crushed amaretti; while in Veneto and Sicily it is mostly served fried in a sweet-and-sour sauce.

I never use large, round pumpkins which have no taste – in my opinion, they are only good for making Halloween lanterns. I prefer to use the smaller butternut squash which is full of flavour and available year round.

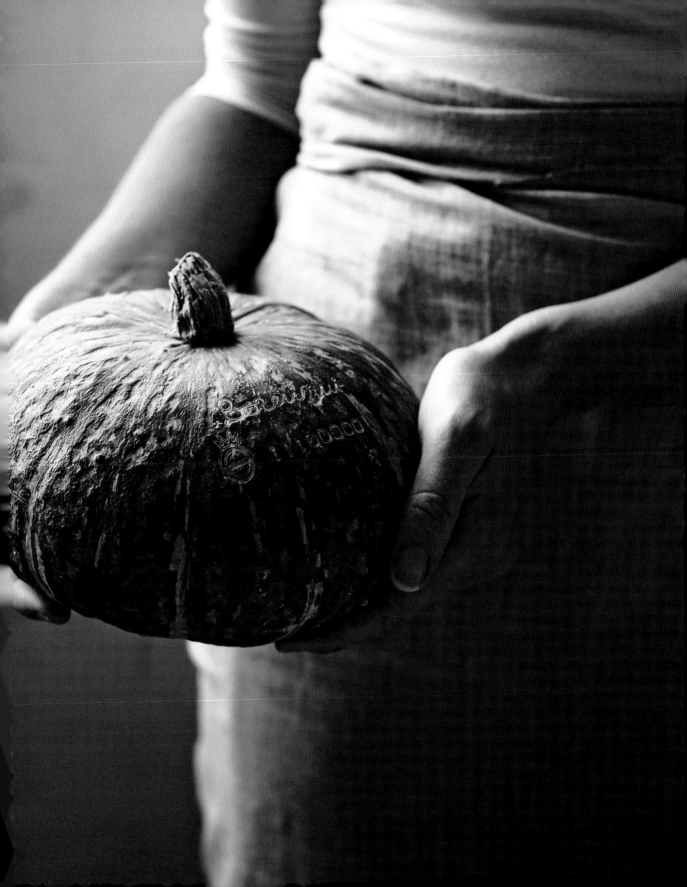

Minestra di Zucca e Cicoria
Butternut Squash and Chicory Soup

This recipe comes from Mantova (Mantua), a town in Lombardy which prides itself on two things: one of the most beautiful palazzi in Italy – Il Palazzo Ducale – and the *zucca mantovana*. I am not qualified to talk about the palazzo, but I can certainly tell you that *zucca mantovana* is the best pumpkin you can have. It is a very large pumpkin with deep yellow pulp covered by bright green skin. When in season in September and October, it is everywhere. It can be cooked in many ways: as a soup, fried and then served in a sweet and sour sauce or used as a filling for ravioli or sweet pies.

In the original recipe the bitterness of the chicory balances the sweetness of the pumpkin. However, I suggest you use butternut squash, which I prefer to pumpkin, and which is easy to find.

Serves 4
250g/9oz butternut squash, peeled
1 chicory
50g/2oz/4 tbsp unsalted butter
½ onion, chopped
1.2 litres/2 pints/5 cups vegetable stock
Sea salt and freshly ground black
*   pepper*
Crostini (see page 199)
Freshly grated Parmesan to serve

Cut the squash into cubes about 3cm/1¼in thick. Cut the chicory in 1cm/½in strips. Wash and drain the chicory.

Melt the butter in a large saucepan and add the onion and a pinch or two of salt. Gently sauté for 7–8 minutes and then add the butternut squash. Sauté for about 5 minutes, turning the cubes over and over in the buttery onion. Add the chicory and do the same with it.

Heat 1 litre/1¾ pints/4 cups of the stock and pour it over the vegetables. Mix well, season with salt and pepper, cover with a lid and bring to the boil. Simmer for 30 minutes or so, until the butternut squash is tender.

Purée the soup either with a stick blender – the easiest – or in a blender or food processor, taste and adjust the seasoning. If you like a thinner soup, add the remaining stock and warm through.

Ladle the soup into individual bowls and hand around the crostini and Parmesan in bowls.

Gnocchi di Zucca
Pumpkin Gnocchi

Butternut or kabocha squash mixed with sweet potatoes comes close to the spicy sweetness and moist texture of a northern Italian pumpkin. These gnocchi are a speciality of Veneto and southern Lombardy. The cinnamon dressing is the classic dressing from Veneto, while the sage dressing from Lombardy is the one that is mostly used everywhere else.

I find it easiest to make these soft pumpkin gnocchi with a piping bag and a plain, large nozzle, but you may prefer to make them the more traditional way, shaping the gnocchi into small balls, using floured hands.

Serves 4–5

1 tbsp vegetable oil

500g/1lb 2oz butternut or kabocha squash

500g/1lb 2oz sweet potatoes

200g/7oz/generous 1 1/2 cups flour

2 tsp baking powder

A good pinch of salt

2 large (US extra-large) eggs

4 tbsp freshly grated Parmesan

A generous grating of nutmeg

For the cinnamon dressing

75g/2 3/4oz/5 tbsp unsalted butter

5 tbsp Parmesan, grated

1 tbsp sugar

1 tsp ground cinnamon

For the sage dressing

75g/2 3/4oz/5 tbsp unsalted butter

6 sage leaves, snipped

10 tbsp Parmesan, grated

Heat the oven to 160°C Fan/180°C/350°F/Gas Mark 4.

Line a baking sheet with foil and brush the foil with oil. Wipe the squash and cut it in half. Scoop out and discard the seeds and fibres and place the squash, cut side down, on the foil. Pierce the sweet potatoes with a skewer and place them on the foil with the squash. Bake for about 1 hour, until both vegetables can be pierced easily with a fork.

Peel the sweet potatoes and scoop the flesh out of the squash. Purée both vegetables through a food mill or a potato ricer into a bowl. Mix in most of the flour, baking powder and a good pinch of salt and then break in the eggs. Mix very well to incorporate, adding a little more flour if necessary until you can gather the dough into a ball, then add the Parmesan and season with nutmeg and salt to taste. If you have time, put the mixture in the refrigerator for 30 minutes or so; it is easier to shape when it is cold.

Bring a large saucepan of salted water to the boil. To pipe the gnocchi, fill the piping bag with the squash mixture and hold it over the saucepan, squeezing it with one hand and cutting the mixture with the other as it comes out of the nozzle. Cut short shapes about 2cm/¾in long, letting them drop straight into the simmering water. Don't cook all the gnocchi together, but do it in three batches. Cook them for 1–2 minutes after they have risen to the surface of the water. Lift out with a slotted spoon and place in a large, shallow ovenproof dish. Spoon a little dressing over each batch and keep the dish warm in a low oven.

For the cinnamon dressing, melt the butter in a bain-marie or double boiler and then pour it over the gnocchi and sprinkle with the Parmesan, sugar and cinnamon.

For the sage dressing, put the butter and sage leaves in a small saucepan and let the butter melt and begin to foam. Spoon over the gnocchi and sprinkle with the Parmesan.

Zucchina
Courgette

Like many other vegetables the courgette arrived from the New World and soon became quite popular in Europe. Many people find courgettes rather tasteless, but they are not; they have a delicate flavour which is sometimes overwhelmed by the addition of ingredients with flavours that are too strong. Courgettes don't need much tweaking: a few leaves of fresh mint, one or two garlic cloves, a little tomato purée or a spoonful or two of a good tomato sauce, a sautéed shallot or a small piece of onion.

In Italy there are many varieties of *zucchine* of different shapes and colours – round and squat, oblong and fat, long and thin, while in Britain the most common courgette is long and green. Occasionally you can find small, round courgettes which are ideal for stuffing: cut off the top, scoop out the seeds and stuff the courgette cup. The stuffing can vary from minced meat or minced chicken to cheese and egg or just breadcrumbs, anchovy fillets and parsley, usually mixed with the pulp of the courgette. My favourite stuffing is made with the pulp of the courgettes, lightly fried in oil to which some crumbled amaretti biscuits and a spoonful or two of ricotta cheese are added at the end.

You can also eat courgette flowers, which should be picked early in the morning when the flower has not yet opened up to the sun. They are one of the most delicious vegetables to eat fried (see page 190), but they also make a good pasta sauce, gently sautéed in butter and finished off with cream and Parmesan cheese.

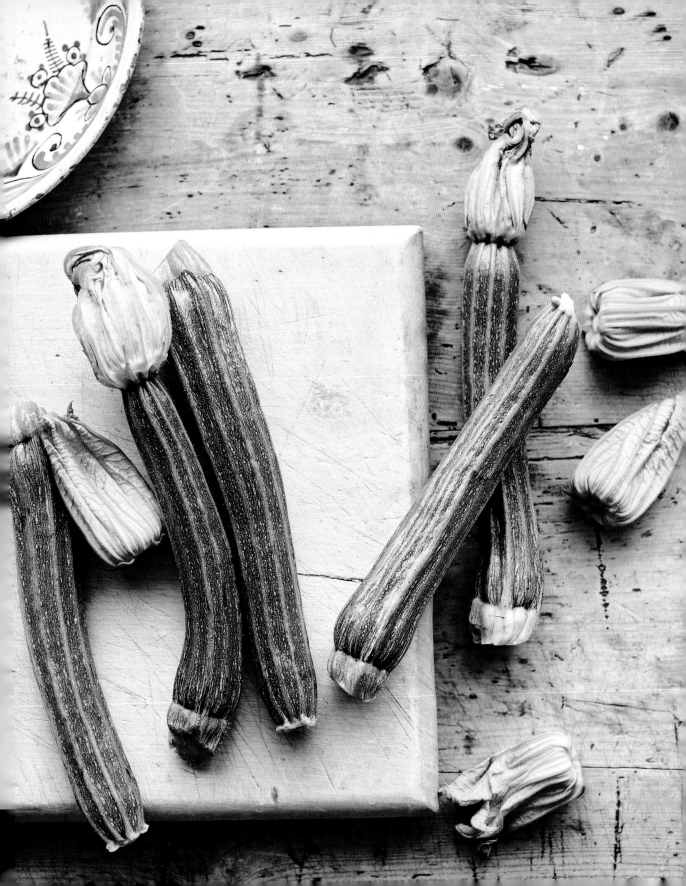

Zucchine al Forno al Sapor di Mentuccia
Baked Courgettes with Mint and Garlic

The ideal courgette for this dish is one about 15cm/6in long. Don't buy very large courgettes, which contain too many watery seeds, nor the baby ones, which have very little flavour.

You can produce a perfect vegetarian course serving these courgettes with *Pomodorini Arrostiti* or Roasted Cherry Tomatoes (see page 137).

Serves 6

6 courgettes (zucchini)

4 tbsp chopped flat leaf parsley

8 tbsp chopped mint leaves

3–4 garlic cloves

8 tbsp dried breadcrumbs

100ml/3½fl oz/7 tbsp extra virgin olive oil

Sea salt and freshly ground black pepper

Wash and dry the courgettes, chop off the two ends and cut the courgettes lengthwise. Sprinkle the cut sides lightly with sea salt and place them on a wooden board, cut side down. Leave them for at least 30 minutes. During this time some of the vegetable liquid will drain away.

Heat the oven to 160°C Fan/180°C/350°F/Gas Mark 4.

To make the stuffing, put the chopped herbs, garlic and breadcrumbs in a bowl and gradually add half the oil, while beating the mixture with a fork. When this is done, season with salt and a generous grinding of pepper.

Brush a baking sheet large enough to hold the courgette halves in a single layer lightly with oil.

Wipe the courgette halves with kitchen paper and lay them, cut side up, on the sheet. Brush the courgettes with a little of the oil and then pile some of the herb mixture over each half. Drizzle with about half the remaining oil and place the tray in the oven. Bake until the courgettes are tender – test by inserting a knife into them – which will be about 20–25 minutes.

Remove from the oven and place two courgette halves on each plate. Drizzle the remaining oil over them and serve warm or at room temperature.

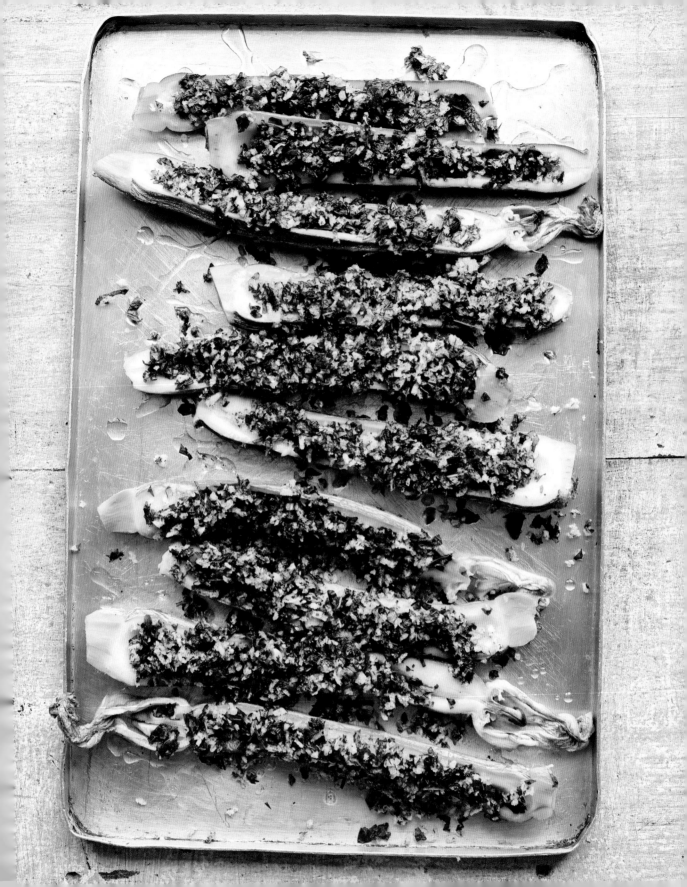

Zucchine alla Umbra
Courgettes with Tomatoes

This recipe is supposed to come from Umbria, but frankly it could come from anywhere in Italy, since it is such an obvious way to cook courgettes. The result is quite delicious.

Serves 4

300g/10½oz cherry tomatoes

500g/1lb 2 oz courgettes (zucchini)

250ml/9fl oz/8½ cups vegetable stock

2 garlic cloves

Sea salt and freshly ground black pepper

2 tbsp extra virgin olive oil

Bring a saucepan of water to the boil. Make a small cut at the bottom of each tomato and add to the pan. Turn the water off and leave the tomatoes in it for about 30–40 seconds. Rinse them under cold water and peel them – the skins should slip off quite easily.

Wash and dry the courgettes. Cut them into 7–8cm/2¾–3¼in chunks and cut the chunks into quarters so that you have thick sticks. Put the courgettes in a sauté pan, add the stock and bring to the boil. Cook for 5 minutes until just beginning to soften.

Cut the garlic cloves in half and remove the hard germ – if there is one. Put the cloves on a chopping board, add the tomatoes and chop to a mush.

Now go back to the courgettes. If there is still some stock in the pan, boil fast to evaporate. Mix in the tomato and garlic mixture and cook until the courgettes are done, which depends on how you like them. I cook them for some 7–8 minutes, but you might like yours more al dente. Season with salt and pepper and stir in the oil. Serve warm or at room temperature.

Passato di Zucchine, Cipolle e Pomodori
Courgette, Onion and Tomato Soup

I owe this soup to my friend Myriam. For health reasons, she is the puréed soup expert par excellence. She is also a very good cook, as you can judge by this delicious soup.

Serves 4

1 tbsp oil

1 onion, finely sliced

25g/1oz/1½ tbsp unsalted butter

4 courgettes (zucchini), cut into thin slices

3 ripe tomatoes, peeled and coarsely chopped

1 litre/1¾ pints/4 cups hot chicken or vegetable stock

Sea salt and freshly ground black pepper

Heat the oil in a sauté pan and add the onion and a pinch or two of salt. Sauté for some 5 minutes, stirring frequently and then add the butter and the courgettes. Sauté over a gentle heat for 5 minutes and then add the tomatoes. Continue cooking for a further 10 minutes. Pour in about 700ml/1¼ pints/3 cups of the stock, cover the pan, bring to the boil and simmer for 15 minutes. Season with pepper, taste and adjust the salt.

Blend the soup with a stick blender – the easiest – in a food processor or a liquidizer. If you like the soup thinner, add some of the remaining hot stock and then ladle the soup into warmed bowls. Serve with crostini (see page 199), if you like.

Insalata di Zucchine, Pomodori e Mozzarella
Courgette, Tomato and Mozzarella Salad

I have a spiralizer machine and I use it for slicing the courgettes for this salad. I love the long curls. But if you don't have a spiralizer, a mandolin works well, too, and it certainly does not make any difference to the deliciousness of this salad.

Buy thin courgettes, as they have fewer seeds than large ones.

Serves 4

4 courgettes (zucchini)

Juice of 1 unwaxed lemon

12 cherry tomatoes

12 buffalo mozzarella balls, cut into
  quarters

4 tbsp extra virgin olive oil

Sea salt and freshly ground black
  pepper

12 basil leaves, torn

Wash and dry the courgettes, then cut them with either a spiralizer or mandoline. Once cut, put the courgettes in a salad bowl and mix in 1 tbsp of lemon juice.

Wash and dry the tomatoes and cut them in half. Add to the salad bowl, along with the mozzarella balls.

Pour the oil into the bowl and toss, using two forks, which are better for separating all the bits. Season with salt and pepper and then taste and adjust both the lemon juice and the seasoning. Before serving, scatter the top of the salad with the basil leaves.

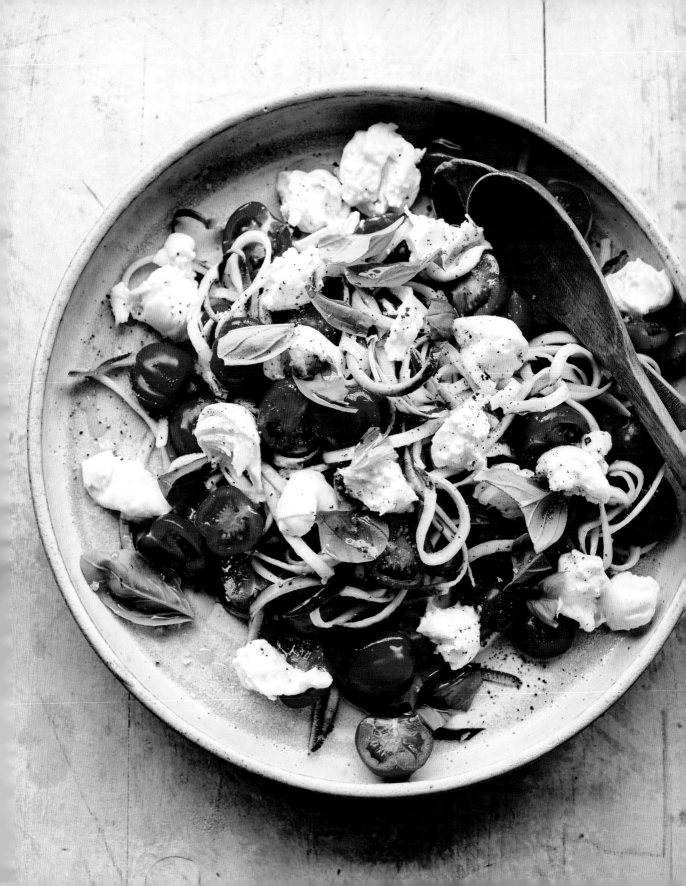

Fiori di Zucca Fritti
Fried Courgette Flowers

This is one of the most delicious dishes I know. Alas, it is not easy to make since the flowers should be just soft and juicy wrapped in a shield of crunchy batter. I have also included an alternative batter using beer and a tasty cheese and anchovy stuffing.

Serves 4

16 large courgette (zucchini) flowers
1.5 litres/2¾ pints/6½ cups sunflower
  oil

For the batter

150g/5oz flour
2 tbsp olive oil
Sea salt
2 egg whites

For the beer batter, optional

100g/3½oz flour
Sea salt and freshly ground black
  pepper
1 egg
150ml/5fl oz/⅔ cup lager beer

For the stuffing, optional

250g/9oz mozzarella, cut into small
  pieces
6 anchovy fillets, drained

Start by making the batter. Using an electric mixer beat together the flour, oil and a pinch or two of salt, while adding 200ml/7fl oz/scant 1 cup of cold water. Beat well, cover the batter and chill for at least 1 hour.

Wipe clean the flowers, open them gently and remove the stamens.

Whisk the egg whites and fold gently into the batter.

Heat the oil to 190°C/375°F. Take a courgette flower by the stem, dip it into the batter and then straight into the hot oil. Repeat with the remaining flowers in batches but do not fry too many at the same time. While they are frying, move them around with a long wooden fork so that they fry evenly. When they are crisp and golden, scoop them out of the oil with a slotted spoon and place them on kitchen paper to drain. Sprinkle with salt and eat them eat straight away.

Fried food should always be eaten immediately. The Neapolitans, famous for their fried food, say, *Frienno e mangianno* or 'fry and eat'.

For the alternative beer batter and stuffing: whisk the flour, seasoning, egg and beer until just blended. Wipe clean the flowers, open them gently and remove the stamens. Fill each flower with about 15g/½oz of mozzarella and a piece of anchovy fillet and gently twist the top to close it. Cook the courgette flowers as above. This should take about 6–8 minutes.

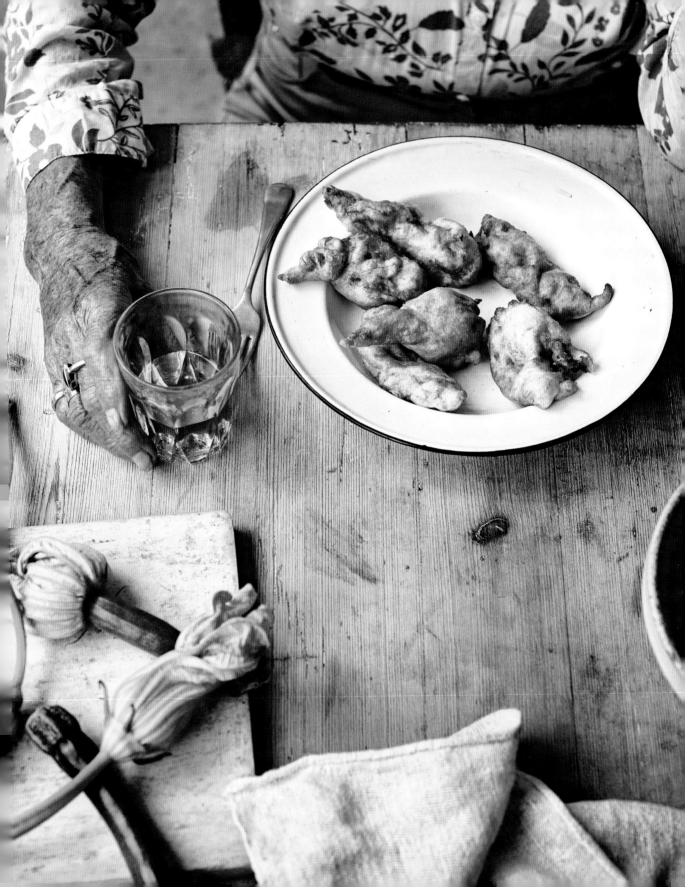

Sauces and mixed vegetable dishes

Right: Aquacotta (see page 202)

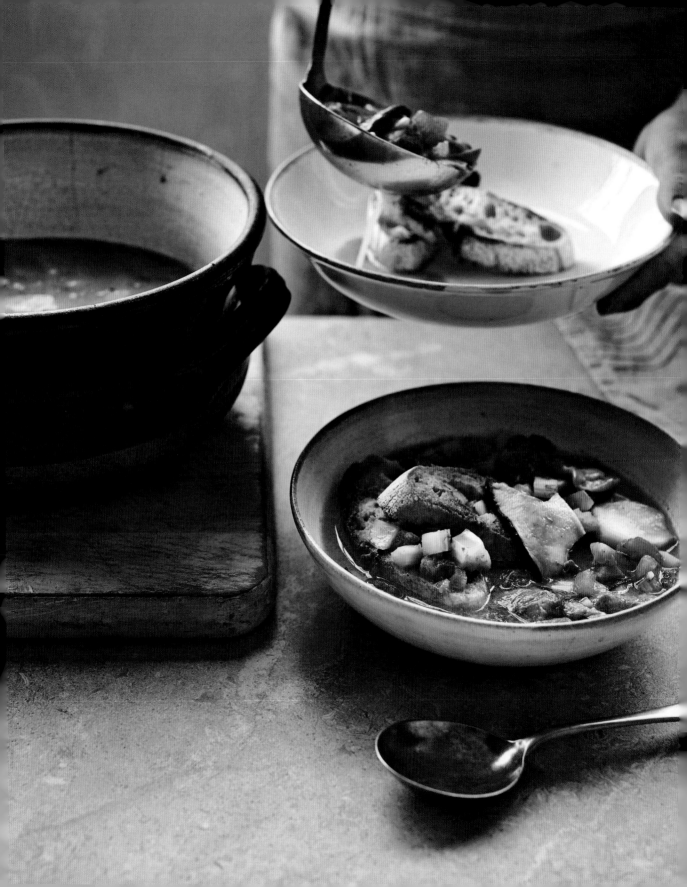

Salsa Verde
Green Sauce

Makes about 150ml/5fl oz/²/₃ cup

15g/¹/₂oz/1 tbsp fresh white
    breadcrumbs

1 tbsp red wine vinegar

1 garlic clove

20g/1oz flat leaf parsley

2 tbsp capers, preferably in salt, rinsed

6 cornichons

1 egg, hard-boiled

4 canned or bottled anchovy fillets,
    drained

2 tsp Dijon mustard

150ml/5fl oz/²/₃ cup extra virgin olive
    oil

Salt and freshly ground black pepper

Salsa verde is now popular everywhere, as indeed it should be. Its origins are in Lombardy where the best parsley used to grow. There and throughout northern Italy it is always served with a bollito misto or boiled meats. But it is perfect also with fish, hard-boiled eggs, tuna, boiled vegetables or rice and even the non-Italian couscous. Here is the classic recipe made with vinegar. The oil should be a sweet olive oil (from Liguria or Marche), not a peppery one. If you want to serve salsa verde with fish, substitute lemon for the vinegar.

Put the breadcrumbs in a bowl, pour the vinegar over and set aside.

Cut the garlic in half and remove the green central germ if necessary. Put the garlic in the bowl of a food processor, together with the parsley, capers, cornichons, hard-boiled egg, anchovy fillets and mustard. Whizz for a few seconds. Squeeze the vinegar out of the breadcrumbs and add the crumbs to the parsley mixture. Start whizzing again while slowly adding the oil through the funnel. Stop occasionally and scoop down all the bits splattered around the bowl. Spoon the sauce into a bowl and add salt and pepper to taste. Feel free to add a little more vinegar if you like a more tart sauce.

Salsa Rossa
Red Sauce

Makes about 200ml/7fl oz/scant 1 cup

500g/1lb 2oz ripe tomatoes, peeled

2 tsp tomato purée (paste)

1 tsp white sugar

1 onion, coarsely chopped

1 carrot, coarsely chopped

1 celery stalk, coarsely chopped

3 garlic cloves

¹/₂ tsp ground cloves

¹/₄ tsp ground cinnamon

3 tbsp extra virgin olive oil

1 tbsp red wine vinegar

Salt and freshly ground black pepper

This tomato sauce is never used for dressing pasta; it is the sauce served in Piedmont with salsa verde (see above) to accompany bollito misto (boiled meats). It is also good with many other foods: fish, hard-boiled eggs, gammon or even boiled potatoes.

Put all the ingredients, except the oil, vinegar, salt and pepper in a heavy-based pan and cook over a low heat for at least 1–1½ hours is even better. Keep an eye on the sauce and add a little water if the sauce is slightly sticking to the bottom of the pan.

Purée the sauce with a stick blender – the easiest – or in a food processor or liquidizer. Return the purée to the pan and add the oil, vinegar and salt and pepper to taste. Cook for a further 30 minutes, always over a low heat. Remember to stir occasionally. Now the sauce is ready. Serve warm or at room temperature.

Gremolada

Makes about 175ml/6fl oz/³/₄ cup
150ml/5fl oz/²/₃ cup beef stock
Grated rind of 1 unwaxed lemon
5 tbsp chopped flat leaf parsley
2 garlic cloves, chopped

This sauce from Lombardy is added to *ossobuco* at the end of the cooking. It really should not appear in this book about vegetables, but I think it is a great little sauce which can flavour many steamed vegetables, such as potatoes, broad beans, carrots, green beans, cannellini or lentils. The ideal stock is diluted gravy from your roasted joint. If you don't have any lurking at the back of the refrigerator, make a strong stock with some beef bouillon.

Heat the stock. Put the lemon rind, parsley and garlic in a bowl and gradually add the stock while beating with a fork. Taste and adjust the seasoning. That's all.

Intingolo di Pomodori Secchi e Peperoni
Sundried Tomato and Pepper Relish

Serves 4
2 large yellow peppers (bell peppers)
2 tbsp extra virgin olive oil
2 shallots, very finely chopped
1 garlic clove, very finely chopped
½ tsp chilli (chili) flakes, or more if you want
Sea salt
100g/3½oz anchovy fillets, drained and chopped
1 tbsp balsamic vinegar
200g/7oz sundried tomatoes, drained and cut into short strips
2 tbsp capers, rinsed

Intingolo – such a lovely sound – is untranslatable. It is a zesty relish eaten with bread and makes an ideal topping for a garlicky crisp bruschetta. Buy the sundried tomatoes in oil, not the ones that need rehydrating.

First grill the peppers. The best way to do this is directly over a flame, rather than under a grill. Put a wire rack on the gas ring and then place the peppers straight on top and leave them until the skin is black. Turn the peppers over and burn another side of the pepper and continue until the whole pepper is blackish. Be careful not to leave the pepper too long in the same position or it will burn through the pulp as well and you will have a hole. If you do not have a direct flame, put the peppers under the grill and turn them over and over until they are charred all over.

Remove the skins using your hands or a small knife. Don't wash the peppers because you will wash away their juices. Wipe the peppers clean with damp kitchen paper, cut them in half and remove the cores and seeds. Cut them into thin strips the same size as the tomatoes.

Heat the oil in a frying pan and add the shallot, garlic, chilli and a pinch or two of salt. Sauté for 5 minutes, stirring frequently and then add the anchovies and vinegar and cook over a low heat for 5 minutes, stirring frequently. Add the tomatoes. Mix well and continue cooking for 5 minutes or so. Add the peppers, mix thoroughly and cook gently for 5 minutes so the flavours can blend together. Mix in the capers, taste and check the salt. Serve with plenty of crusty bread or spread over slices of bruschetta.

Pesto
Basil Sauce

Makes about 200ml/7fl oz/scant 1 cup
20g/³⁄₄oz/2¹⁄₂ tbsp pine nuts
60g/2¹⁄₄oz basil leaves
1 garlic clove
125ml/4fl oz/¹⁄₂ cup extra virgin olive
*   oil, preferably Ligurian or from*
*   Le Marche*
4 tbsp freshly grated Parmesan
2 tbsp freshly grated mature pecorino
Sea salt

Until well after the Second World War pesto was unknown outside its home region of Liguria. My mother prided herself on her pesto, which she made while we were spending our summer holidays on the Riviera. Jars and jars of pesto were prepared there, sealed and packed to keep us happy during the grey winter months back in Lombardy. Eating it brought back memories of sun, sea, figs, olives and all the things we loved. The pesto of the western Riviera contains more garlic and often no pine nuts – it is slightly coarser, similar to the Provençal *pistou*; the eastern Riviera version is more delicate and is often finished with a knob of butter. Use a light olive oil and fresh nuts.

Dry fry the pine nuts in a small frying pan for a few minutes, until they release their aroma, being careful not to let them burn. When they are golden, tip them into a food processor or blender with the basil and the garlic. Pulse the machine for a few seconds and then gradually add the oil through the funnel. Scoop the mixture into a bowl and mix in the cheeses and salt to taste.

Pesto di Rucola
Rocket Pesto

Makes about 200ml/7fl oz/scant 1 cup
50g/1³⁄₄oz/6 tbsp pine nuts
100g/3¹⁄₂oz rocket (arugula)
1 garlic clove
Sea salt and freshly ground black
*   pepper*
125ml/4fl oz/¹⁄₂ cup extra virgin
*   olive oil*
50g/1³⁄₄oz pecorino, grated

Pesto sauces of different ingredients are very quick to make and very good to eat. This is a relatively new variation, which can be made all the year round now that rocket leaves are always available. You can make it half and half with rocket and parsley if you want a milder sauce. Spread it on tomatoes cut in half or on hard-boiled eggs, also cut in half.

Dry fry the pine nuts in a small frying pan for a few minutes, until they release their aroma, being careful not to let them burn. When they are golden, tip them into a food processor or blender.

Add the rocket, garlic, salt and pepper to taste and 4 tbsp of the oil and blitz while you add the remaining oil through the funnel until everything is well blended. Taste and adjust the seasoning, then spoon the pesto into a serving bowl. Mix in the pecorino.

Right: Pesto di Rucola

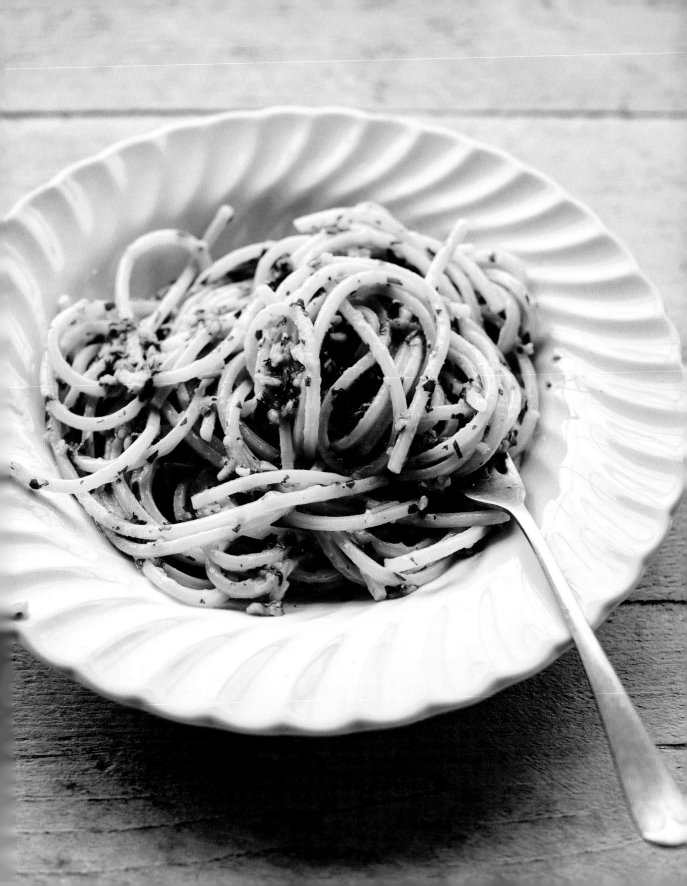

Insalata Russa
Russian Salad

Nobody really knows why this salad is called Russian. Apparently in Russia a similar salad is called an Italian salad. In Italy it is one of the most popular cold dishes you can find in any delicatessen or on any restaurant trolley. It can be surrounded by prawns, imperially topped by half a lobster or modestly decorated with pieces of ox tongue or hard-boiled eggs. In my home in Milan, my mother used to make *Insalata Russa* quite often as an antipasto for her dinner parties and so did I when I used to have dinner parties. The same recipe, the same success. And here it is – the Del Conte senior original.

You can use a good brand of ready made mayonnaise, if you prefer – you will need about 200ml/7fl oz/scant 1 cup – to which you need to add 1 tbsp of lemon juice. Sometimes jars of French cornichons include a few small pickled onions; if you see any like this, buy them – they are good – and use some of the onions in the salad, too.

Serves 4–5

200g/7oz waxy potatoes, scrubbed

125g/4½oz carrots, peeled

200g/7oz cauliflower, outer leaves and stalk removed, cut into small florets

125g/4½oz green beans, topped and tailed and washed

100g/3½oz shelled fresh peas or frozen peas, thawed and drained

50g/1¾oz gherkins, cut into small pieces

2 tbsp small capers, rinsed

200ml/7fl oz/scant 1 cup mayonnaise (see below)

1 tsp English mustard powder

2 tbsp extra virgin olive oil

4 anchovy fillets, drained and chopped

Juice of ½ unwaxed lemon

Sea salt and freshly ground black pepper

2 tbsp chopped flat leaf parsley

A few blade of chives, very thinly cut

For the mayonnaise

2 egg yolks

180ml/6fl oz/¾ cup olive oil

Juice of ½ unwaxed lemon

Cook the potatoes in a pan of boiling, salted water. Drain and, when cool enough to handle, peel them.

Cook the carrots in a second saucepan. When tender, lift them out with a slotted spoon and add the cauliflower florets to the pan. Cook until done and then do the same with the beans and the peas.

Cut the potatoes and carrots into small cubes and the beans into short pieces. Put all the vegetables in a bowl and mix in the gherkins and capers. Now the vegetables are prepared, you can make the dressing.

If making the mayonnaise from scratch, place the egg yolks in a bowl and beat together with a wooden spoon or with an electric beater set at a medium speed. Add a little salt and beat again until pale. Add the oil, drop by drop, beating all the time, until the mixture is the consistency of double (heavy) cream. Still beating, add a drop of lemon juice to thin the mixture a little. Continue to add oil and lemon juice until well incorporated and you have a thick, glosssy mayonnaise.

Sprinkle the mustard into the mayonnaise and beat in the olive oil. Add the anchovy fillets and lemon juice and mix well. Gradually spoon about three-quarters of the dressing over the vegetables and mix thoroughly, but gently. Season with pepper and check the salt and lemon juice – you might like to add a little more.

Transfer the salad to a round dish and spread the remaining dressing over. Sprinkle the mound with the chopped herbs.

You can scatter some prawns over and round the salad, or some hard-boiled quail's eggs or cherry tomatoes; they all go very well with the Russian salad.

Verdure Arrostite
Roasted Vegetables

This is the recipe I use for my summer roasted vegetable dish; in the winter I make it with potatoes, squash, carrots and onions.

Serves 4

2 yellow and red peppers (bell peppers)
2 courgettes (zucchini)
1 aubergine (eggplant)
1 red onion, sliced
6 tbsp extra virgin olive oil
225g/8oz passata (strained tomatoes)
25g/1oz/1 cup marjoram leaves,
*   chopped*
25g/1oz/1 cup flat leaf parsley,
*   chopped*
2 garlic cloves, chopped
½ tsp chilli (chili) flakes
Sea salt and freshly ground black
*   pepper*

Heat the oven to 160°C Fan/180°C/350°F/Gas Mark 4.

Wash and dry the peppers, cut them in half, scrape away the cores, seeds and ribs and cut the halves in half again. Wash and dry the courgettes and cut them lengthwise into slices, about 5cm/2in thick. Do the same with the aubergine.

Brush a baking sheet lightly with some oil. Spread 1 tbsp of passata across the bottom. Sprinkle with a little of the marjoram and parsley and a touch of garlic and season with salt and pepper. Place the courgette slices along one side of the sheet, followed by the aubergine slices, and then the pepper strips. Scatter the onion, remaining herbs and garlic and the chilli over the vegetables. Roughly spread the remaining passata over and top the whole thing with a shower of the remaining oil and a good seasoning of salt and pepper.

Bake until soft, which takes longer than you think – about 1½ hours. Oddly enough, it is the courgettes which take the longest to cook and, of course, the onion, which becomes soft and juicy after all that time. You can serve it either hot, but not straight from the oven, or warm or at room temperature.

Crostini
Croutons

Crostini are made with white bread because it has less flavour than wholemeal. For the same reason they are never dressed with herbs, garlic or Parmesan. They will keep in an airtight container for 3–4 days and also freeze well. Use 2-day old bread if possible.

Serves 4

200g/7oz good-quality compact bread,
*   such as sourdough, crusts removed*
3 tbsp olive oil

Heat the oven to 180°C Fan/200°C/400°F/Gas Mark 6.

Cut the bread into 2–3cm/¾–1¼in slices and then each slice into 2–3cm/¾–1¼in cubes. Put the oil in a bowl, add the bread and mix around in the oil. Spread them in a single layer on a baking sheet and bake them for 10 minutes, shaking the baking sheet once or twice during the time.

Farro con Verdure
Farro with Mixed Vegetables

Farro is a very nutritious cereal and here, combined with vegetables, it makes a perfect one-dish course. The roasting of the tomatoes brings out their flavour.

Serves 4

250g/9oz small tomatoes

150ml/5fl oz/²/₃ cup extra virgin olive oil

2 large red peppers (bell peppers)

200g/7oz farro

4 celery stalks, about 225g/8oz, strings removed, washed, trimmed and cut into small pieces

250g/9oz carrots, scraped or peeled and cut into discs

2 red onions, about 300g/10½oz, finely chopped

2 garlic cloves, germ removed and chopped

Sea salt and freshly ground black pepper

25g/1oz/1 cup flat leaf parsley, chopped

Heat the oven to 140°C Fan/160°C/325°F/Gas Mark 3.

Wash and dry the tomatoes and cut them in half. Brush a baking sheet with a little of the olive oil and place the tomatoes on it, cut side up. Sprinkle with a little salt and roast for about 20 minutes.

Meanwhile, wash and cut the peppers in half, remove the seeds, cores and ribs, cut into quarters and then into small pieces.

Rinse the farro, put it into a pan, cover with water and bring to the boil. Add 1 tbsp of salt and simmer for about 20–30 minutes until cooked. Drain, transfer to a large serving dish and mix in 1 tbsp of the oil.

In a large sauté pan, heat the rest of the oil. Add the celery, carrots and onions and sauté for 15 minutes. Mix in the peppers and garlic and continue cooking for a further 10 minutes. Add the tomatoes and cook gently for 10 minutes. Season with salt and pepper to taste.

Scoop all the vegetables and their juices into the dish with the farro, mix well, sprinkle with parsley and serve. I think the salad is better served either warm or at room temperature, not straight from the heat.

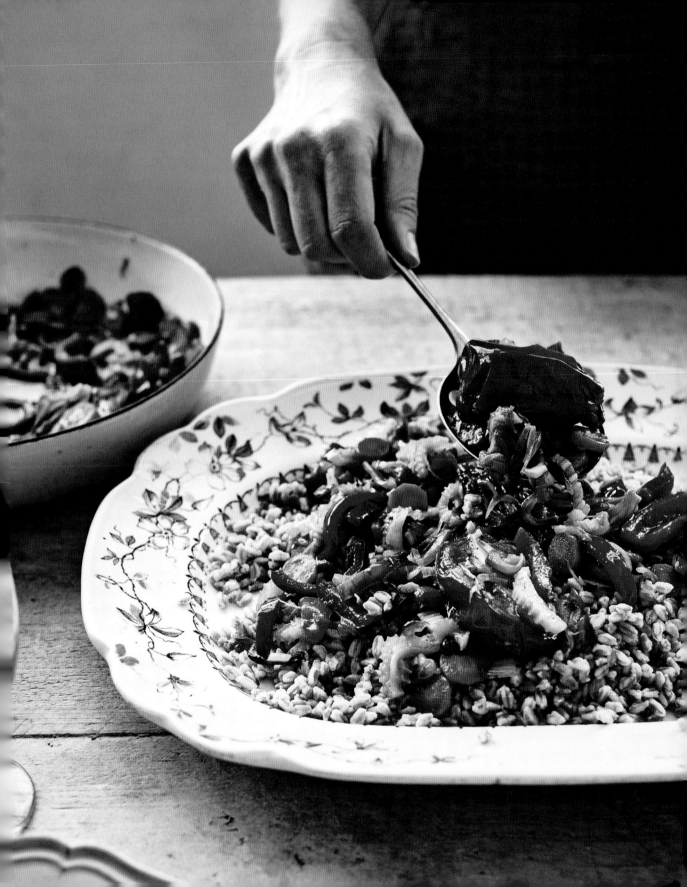

Aquacotta
Vegetable Soup

Acquacotta is a traditional soup of Tuscany. The version here, which I rate the best, is from the provinces of Grosseto and Arezzo and contains fresh porcini. This is one of the few soups that is seasonal, but it is also delicious. I do not think it is worth making the soup with cultivated mushrooms, because they lack the intense earthy flavour necessary for this soup.

If you go mushroom hunting and come home with a basket full of mushrooms – lucky you – you can make this soup with any of the wild varieties, such as parasols, field mushrooms, morels, edible russula, ink caps, chanterelles, puffballs and more as long as you know your mushrooms and leave alone the poisonous ones. Actually there are very few lethal mushrooms, but many are toxic or and totally tasteless and are not worth the trouble of cleaning and eating.

Serves 4

350g/12oz fresh porcini

5 tbsp extra virgin olive oil

2 garlic cloves, chopped

Salt

*250g/9oz fresh ripe tomatoes, skinned
    and chopped*

*4 celery stalks, strings removed and cut
    into small chunks*

Freshly ground black pepper

8 slices of ciabatta

3 large (US extra-large) eggs

3 tbsp freshly grated Parmesan

Clean the porcini, gently scraping the stalks to remove any earth. Wipe them clean with damp kitchen paper and then slice them. If the porcini are large, cut the caps in half before you slice them.

Put 4 tbsp of the oil in a stockpot, together with the porcini, garlic and 1 tsp of salt. Cook for 5 minutes on a medium heat, gently stirring frequently and then add the tomatoes and celery. Sauté gently for a further 10 minutes or so, then pour in 1 litre/1¾ pints/4 cups of hot water. Bring to the boil and turn the heat down so the soup just simmers gently. Simmer for 20 minutes. Taste and season with salt and pepper if required.

Meanwhile, brush the ciabatta slices with the remaining oil and grill the slices on both sides until just slightly golden. Place 2 slices of bread in each individual bowl.

Lightly beat together the eggs with the Parmesan and a pinch of salt. Spoon this mixture into a soup tureen and pour the hot soup over it. Mix well and then ladle the soup over the ciabatta slices in each bowl.

See image on page 193

Minestrone alla Milanese
Minestrone with Rice

There are two traditional *minestroni*: one from Milan – *alla milanese* – and a lighter, fresher version from Genova – *alla genovese*. The Genovese one is made with pasta and is always finished off with a tablespoon of pesto. It is also made with olive oil and not with pancetta, which is an essential part of the Milanese version made with the local rice. This was the minestrone of my childhood in Milan. My father, in his eating habits, was a real Lombard peasant and our weekly minestrone had to be *alla milanese*, apart from during our summer holidays on the coast in Liguria, when he willingly accepted the Genovese version.

I expect that every cook in Lombardy has her or his way to make minestrone. This is mine, my mother's actually, as she and our cook, Maria, used to make it some 80 years ago. The only difference is that the vegetables then were far tastier. But that is another story. Use fresh borlotti beans if you can get hold of them. I always add a piece of pork rind, which gives the soup a particularly rich flavour. When you make minestrone, you might as well make plenty, as it tastes even better reheated.

Serves 8

2 celery stalks, strings removed

2 carrots

500g/1lb 2oz ripe tomatoes

2 courgettes (zucchini)

½ Savoy cabbage

3 medium-size floury (starchy) potatoes

1 large onion

2 garlic cloves

25g/1oz/1 cup flat leaf parsley

6 sage leaves

25g/1oz/2 tbsp unsalted butter

1 tbsp olive oil

100g/3½oz unsmoked pancetta cubes

Piece of pork rind, optional

200g/7oz shelled fresh peas or frozen
    peas, thawed and drained

1 x 400g/14oz can borlotti beans,
    drained and rinsed

Salt and freshly ground black pepper

200g/7oz/1 cup arborio rice

Freshly grated Parmesan to serve

Prepare the vegetables: trim, wash and slice the celery thinly, scrape the carrots and cut into small cubes, peel, deseed and chop the tomatoes and wash and cut the courgettes into small cubes. Wash and cut the cabbage into thick strips and peel the potatoes.

Now prepare the *battuto*: chop together the onion, garlic, parsely and sage. Heat the butter and oil in large saucepan and add the *battuto*, pancetta and pork rind, sauté for some 7–8 minutes, turning the whole thing over frequently and then add the celery, carrots, tomatoes and courgettes and sauté for 2–3 minutes. Now add the potatoes and 3 litres/5¼ pints/12 cups of water. Cover the pan with the lid and cook gently for 2 hours. By the end of cooking the potatoes should have partly disintegrated. Just press them down with a fork to break them up completely so that they thicken the soup.

Add the peas, Savoy cabbage, borlotti beans, and salt and pepper and bring the soup back to the boil. Now add the rice and cook for 15–20 minutes until the rice is done. This soup should be very thick, but you might need to add some boiling water before adding the rice.

When the rice is cooked, fish out the pork rind if you have used one and then ladle the soup into individual bowls and sprinkle with Parmesan. Serve with more Parmesan on the side.

In summer minestrone is also served at room temperature and it is delicious.

A

anchovies: cauliflower salad with
   anchovies 40
   cauliflower with sautéed breadcrumbs
      43
   fried courgette flowers 190
   green beans and Swiss chard cake 76
   green sauce 194
   grilled peppers with anchovies, olives
      and capers 124
   grilled radicchio and chicory 150
   hot garlic and anchovy dip for raw
      vegetables 30
   lamb's lettuce, rocket and pine nut
      salad 97
   puntarelle salad 146
   tomatoes stuffed with rice, anchovies
      and capers 140
artichokes *see* globe artichokes;
   Jerusalem artichokes
arugula *see* rocket
asparagus 13–15
   asparagus with eggs and grated
      Parmesan 14
   baked asparagus wrapped in prosciutto
      16
aubergines (eggplants) 103–11
   aubergine parmigiana 106
   aubergine pizzas 110
   aubergines in a sweet and sour sauce
      111
   aubergines stuffed with bread and
      tomatoes 108
   aubergines with a hundred flavours 104
   celeriac and aubergine braised in
      tomato sauce 161
   fried breaded aubergines 107
   lentils in ratatouille 102
   roasted vegetables 199

B

bacon: leeks in a vinaigrette sauce 145
   see also pancetta
barley *see* pearl barley
basil: pesto 74, 196
beans 77–85
   see also broad beans, cannellini beans
      etc
béchamel sauce 44, 162
beer batter 190
beetroot 17–21
   beetroot gnocchi 21
   beetroot, potato and shallot salad 18
   sautéed beetroot with herbs and garlic
      20

bell peppers *see* peppers
black salsify 156
   black salsify with egg and lemon 156
borlotti bean soup 85
bread and breadcrumbs: aubergines
      stuffed with bread and tomatoes 108
   Brussels sprouts bake 48
   cauliflower with sautéed breadcrumbs
      43
   celery soup 159
   croutons 199
   fried breaded aubergines 107
   pointed cabbage and bread soup 57
   potato cake with mozzarella and
      prosciutto 116
   tomato bruschetta 137
   tomato, spring onion, cucumber and
      crouton salad 138
   vegetable soup 202
broad (fava) beans 77
   broad bean purée with radicchio and
      spring onions 80
   broad bean soup 84
   broad beans with burrata 82
   broad beans with cured pig jowl 83
broccoletti 22
   broccoletti with pulses 24
   broccoletti with tomatoes and spring
      onions 23
broccoli 22–5
   sautéed broccoli with pancetta 23
bruschetta, tomato 137
Brussels sprouts 46–8
   Brussels sprouts bake 48
   roasted Brussels sprouts with rosemary,
      lemon and pecorino 47
butter 8
butternut squash and chicory soup 180

C

cabbage 49–58
   minestrone with rice 203
   pointed cabbage and bread soup 57
   red cabbage cooked in wine 50
   sautéed spiced cabbage 52
   Savoy cabbage and lamb soup 58
   Savoy cabbage stewed with sausages
      51
   see also cavolo nero
cannellini beans: broccoletti with pulses
      24
   cannellini beans and tuna salad 78
   cannellini beans sautéed in garlic oil
      79
   spinach and watercress soup 172

Tuscan cavolo nero soup 56
capers: aubergines in a sweet and sour
      sauce 111
   green sauce 194
   grilled peppers with anchovies, olives
      and capers 124
   tomatoes stuffed with rice, anchovies
      and capers 140
cardoons 30–1
carrots 32–7
   carrot, celeriac and walnut salad 36
   carrot soup 34
   carrots braised in Marsala 34
   carrots in sweet and sour sauce 33
   carrots sautéed in butter 33
   farro with mixed vegetables 200
cauliflower 38–45
   cauliflower and pea bake 44
   cauliflower and potatoes braised in
      tomato sauce 40
   cauliflower salad with anchovies 40
   cauliflower stewed in wine 42
   cauliflower with sautéed breadcrumbs
      43
   Russian salad 198
cavolo nero: cavolo nero and potatoes
      sautéed with chilli and garlic 54
   Tuscan cavolo nero soup 56
celeriac 160–2
   carrot, celeriac and walnut salad 36
   celeriac and aubergine braised in
      tomato sauce 161
   celeriac and spinach bake 162
celery 157–9
   aubergines in a sweet and sour sauce
      111
   celery, Gorgonzola and walnut salad
      158
   celery soup 159
chard *see* Swiss chard
cheese: asparagus with eggs and grated
      Parmesan 14
   aubergine parmigiana 106
   aubergine pizzas 110
   baked fennel 87
   baked onion frittata 66
   broad beans with burrata 82
   Brussels sprouts bake 48
   cauliflower and pea bake 44
   celery, Gorgonzola and walnut salad
      158
   celery soup 159
   courgette, tomato and mozzarella salad
      188
   fennel braised in milk 90

204

fennel, mushroom and pecorino salad 88

fried breaded aubergines 107

fried courgette flowers 190

green bean, ham and Grana Padano salad 72

green beans and Swiss chard cake 76

leek and rice bake 142

leeks baked with cream and cheese 144

mangetout with cream and Parmesan cheese 176

peppers stuffed with goat's cheese and pesto 128

pesto 196

potato and courgette bake 121

potato cake with mozzarella and prosciutto 116

spinach and ricotta gnocchi 167

spinach mould 164

spinach roll 168–70

spinach soup 171

stracciatella with peas 134

Swiss chard bake 70

chickpeas 59–61

  broccoletti with pulses 24

  chickpea and farro soup 60

  sautéed chickpeas and tomatoes 59

chicory: butternut squash and chicory soup 180

  grilled radicchio and chicory 150

chillies 8

  cavolo nero and potatoes sautéed with chilli and garlic 54

  sautéed chickpeas and tomatoes 59

cinnamon dressing 181

cooking times 9

cornichons: green sauce 194

courgette flowers, fried 190

courgettes (zucchini) 182–91

  baked courgettes with mint and garlic 184

  courgette, onion and tomato soup 187

  courgette, tomato and mozzarella salad 188

  courgettes with tomatoes 186

  lentils in ratatouille 102

  potato and courgette bake 121

  roasted vegetables 199

  sautéed potato and courgette sticks 114

croutons 199

cucumber 62

  cucumber, spring onion and purslane salad 62

  radish and cucumber salad 155

  tomato, spring onion, cucumber and crouton salad 138

D

dip, hot garlic and anchovy 30

E

eggplant see aubergines

eggs 8

  asparagus with eggs and grated Parmesan 14

  baked onion frittata 66

  black salsify with egg and lemon 156

  celery soup 159

  potato and courgette bake 121

  roasted peppers with hard-boiled eggs 126

  Swiss chard bake 70

  vegetable soup 202

endive (frisée): red radicchio, endive and orange salad 149

F

farro: chickpea and farro soup 60

  farro with mixed vegetables 200

fava beans see broad beans

fennel, Florence 86–91

  baked fennel 87

  fennel, blood orange and black olive salad 90

  fennel braised in milk 90

  fennel cooked in wine 87

  fennel, mushroom and pecorino salad 88

  red radicchio, endive and orange salad 149

fennel seeds: green beans in fennel-flavoured tomato sauce 73

Florence fennel see fennel, Florence

frisée see endive

frittata, baked onion 66

G

garlic 10–13

  cannellini beans sautéed in garlic oil 79

  cavolo nero and potatoes sautéed with chilli and garlic 54

  garlic sauce 12

  hot garlic and anchovy dip for raw vegetables 30

globe artichokes 26–9

  artichokes and peas 27

  baked artichokes with herbs 28

gnocchi: beetroot gnocchi 21

  pumpkin gnocchi 181

  spinach and ricotta gnocchi 167

goat's cheese: peppers stuffed with goat's cheese and pesto 128

green beans 71–6

  green bean, ham and Grana Padano salad 72

  green beans and potatoes with pesto 74

  green beans and Swiss chard cake 76

  green beans in fennel-flavoured tomato sauce 73

green salad 96

green sauce 194

guanciale: broad beans with cured pig jowl 83

H

ham: green bean, ham and Grana Padano salad 72

J

Jerusalem artichokes 177

  Jerusalem artichoke soup 177

L

lamb: Savoy cabbage and lamb soup 58

  stock 58

lamb's lettuce, rocket and pine nut salad 97

leeks 141–5

  green beans and Swiss chard cake 76

  leek and rice bake 142

  leeks baked with cream and cheese 144

  leeks in a vinaigrette sauce 145

  Tuscan cavolo nero soup 56

lemon 8

  black salsify with egg and lemon 156

  gremolada 195

  roasted Brussels sprouts with rosemary, lemon and pecorino 47

lentils 98–102

  broccoletti with pulses 24

  lentil soup 99

  lentils in ratatouille 102

  stewed lentils with sundried tomatoes 100

lettuce 95–7

  green salad 96

  lamb's lettuce, rocket and pine nut salad 97

M

mangetout 175–6

mangetout with cream and Parmesan
cheese 176
Marsala, carrots braised in 34
milk, fennel braised in 90
minestrone with rice 203
mushrooms 8, 92–4
fennel, mushroom and pecorino salad
88
peas and mushrooms with marjoram
133
sautéed mushrooms 93
vegetable soup 202
wild mushroom and pearl barley soup
94

O

olive oil 9
olives: aubergines in a sweet and sour
sauce 111
fennel, blood orange and black olive
salad 90
grilled peppers with anchovies, olives
and capers 124
onions 63–9
baked onion frittata 66
courgette, onion and tomato soup 187
onion soup 69
onions stuffed with tuna 64
small onions in sweet and sour sauce
68
see also spring onions
oranges: fennel, blood orange and black
olive salad 90
red radicchio, endive and orange salad
149

P

pancetta 9
borlotti bean soup 85
sautéed broccoli with pancetta 23
stewed lentils with sundried tomatoes
100
parsley: gremolada 195
pasta: borlotti bean soup 85
pearl barley: wild mushroom and pearl
barley soup 94
pears: pea and pear soup 135
peas 130–5
artichokes and peas 27
broccoletti with pulses 24
cauliflower and pea bake 44
minestrone with rice 203
pea and pear soup 135
peas and mushrooms with marjoram
133

peas with prosciutto 131
peas with tarragon 132
stracciatella with peas 134
pepper 9
peppers (bell peppers) 122–9
farro with mixed vegetables 200
grilled peppers with anchovies, olives
and capers 124
lentils in ratatouille 102
pepper and tomato ratatouille 129
peppers in a vinegary sauce 125
peppers stuffed with goat's cheese and
pesto 128
roasted peppers with hard-boiled eggs
126
roasted vegetables 199
sundried tomato and pepper relish 195
pesto 196
green beans and potatoes with pesto 74
peppers stuffed with goat's cheese and
pesto 128
rocket pesto 196
pine nuts: lamb's lettuce, rocket and pine
nut salad 97
pesto 196
rocket pesto 196
spinach with sultanas and pine nuts
166
pizzas, aubergine 110
pointed cabbage and bread soup 57
porcini 8
sautéed mushrooms 93
vegetable soup 202
pork: broad beans with cured pig jowl 83
potatoes 112–21
baked artichokes with herbs 28
baked potato cakes 118
beetroot gnocchi 21
beetroot, potato and shallot salad 18
broad bean purée with radicchio and
spring onions 80
cauliflower and potatoes braised in
tomato sauce 40
cavolo nero and potatoes sautéed with
chilli and garlic 54
green beans and potatoes with pesto
74
mashed potatoes 120
potato and courgette bake 121
potato cake with mozzarella and
prosciutto 116
potato gnocchi 117
Russian salad 198
sautéed potato and courgette sticks 114
sautéed potatoes with parsley and

garlic 115
spinach roll 168–70
warm potato salad with chilli 113
prosciutto 9
baked asparagus wrapped in prosciutto
16
peas with prosciutto 131
potato cake with mozzarella and
prosciutto 116
pulses see beans; chickpeas; lentils
pumpkin 178
pumpkin gnocchi 181
puntarelle 146
puntarelle salad 146
purslane: cucumber, spring onion and
purslane salad 62

R

radicchio 148–51
broad bean purée with radicchio and
spring onions 80
grilled radicchio and chicory 150
red radicchio, endive and orange salad
149
radishes 154–5
radish and cucumber salad 155
ratatouille: lentils in ratatouille 102
pepper and tomato ratatouille 129
red cabbage cooked in wine 50
red sauce 194
relish, sundried tomato and pepper 195
rice: Jerusalem artichoke soup 177
leek and rice bake 142
minestrone with rice 203
tomatoes stuffed with rice, anchovies
and capers 140
roasted vegetables 199
rocket (arugula): lamb's lettuce, rocket
and pine nut salad 97
rocket pesto 196
Russian salad 198

S

sage dressing 181
salads: beetroot, potato and shallot salad
18
cannellini beans and tuna salad 78
carrot, celeriac and walnut salad 36
cauliflower salad with anchovies 40
celery, Gorgonzola and walnut salad
158
courgette, tomato and mozzarella
salad 188
cucumber, spring onion and purslane
salad 62

fennel, blood orange and black olive salad 90
fennel, mushroom and pecorino salad 88
green bean, ham and Grana Padano salad 72
green salad 96
lamb's lettuce, rocket and pine nut salad 97
puntarelle salad 146
radish and cucumber salad 155
red radicchio, endive and orange salad 149
Russian salad 198
tomato, spring onion, cucumber and crouton salad 138
warm potato salad with chilli 113
salsify *see* black salsify
salt 9
sauces: béchamel sauce 44, 162
  garlic sauce 12
  green sauce 194
  pesto 74, 196
  red sauce 194
  rocket pesto 196
  tomato sauce 110
sausages: celery soup 159
  Savoy cabbage stewed with sausages 51
Savoy cabbage and lamb soup 58
Savoy cabbage stewed with sausages 51
scallions *see* spring onions
soffritto: chickpea and farro soup 60
soups: borlotti bean soup 85
  broad bean soup 84
  butternut squash and chicory soup 180
  carrot soup 34
  celery soup 159
  chickpea and farro soup 60
  courgette, onion and tomato soup 187
  Jerusalem artichoke soup 177
  lentil soup 99
  minestrone with rice 203
  onion soup 69
  pea and pear soup 135
  pointed cabbage and bread soup 57
  Savoy cabbage and lamb soup 58
  spinach and watercress soup 172
  spinach soup 171
  stracciatella with peas 134
  Tuscan cavolo nero soup 56
  vegetable soup 202
  wild mushroom and pearl barley soup 94
spinach 163–74

celeriac and spinach bake 162
spinach and ricotta gnocchi 167
spinach and watercress soup 172
spinach cake from Lombardy 174
spinach mould 164
spinach roll 168–70
spinach soup 171
spinach with sultanas and pine nuts 166
spring onions (scallions): broad bean purée with radicchio and spring onions 80
  broccoletti with tomatoes and spring onions 23
  cucumber, spring onion and purslane salad 62
  tomato, spring onion, cucumber and crouton salad 138
squash 178–81
  butternut squash and chicory soup 180
  pumpkin gnocchi 181
stewed lentils with sundried tomatoes 100
stock 9
  lamb stock 58
sultanas (golden raisins): aubergines with a hundred flavours 104
  spinach with sultanas and pine nuts 166
sundried tomato and pepper relish 195
sweet and sour sauce: aubergines in 111
  carrots in 33
  small onions in 68
sweet potatoes: pumpkin gnocchi 181
Swiss chard 69–70
  green beans and Swiss chard cake 76
  Swiss chard bake 70
  Swiss chard in tomato sauce 70

T
tipsy cauliflower 42
tipsy fennel 87
tipsy red cabbage 50
tomatoes 9, 136–40
  aubergine parmigiana 106
  aubergine pizzas 110
  aubergines in a sweet and sour sauce 111
  aubergines stuffed with bread and tomatoes 108
  broad bean soup 84
  broccoletti with pulses 24
  broccoletti with tomatoes and spring onions 23
  cauliflower and potatoes braised in

tomato sauce 40
  celeriac and aubergine braised in tomato sauce 161
  courgette, onion and tomato soup 187
  courgette, tomato and mozzarella salad 188
  courgettes with tomatoes 186
  farro with mixed vegetables 200
  green beans in fennel-flavoured tomato sauce 73
  lentil soup 99
  lentils in ratatouille 102
  minestrone with rice 203
  onion soup 69
  pepper and tomato ratatouille 129
  red sauce 194
  roasted cherry tomatoes 137
  roasted vegetables 199
  sautéed chickpeas and tomatoes 59
  stewed lentils with sundried tomatoes 100
  sundried tomato and pepper relish 195
  Swiss chard in tomato sauce 70
  tomato bruschetta 137
  tomato, spring onion, cucumber and crouton salad 138
  tomatoes stuffed with rice, anchovies and capers 140
  Tuscan cavolo nero soup 56
  vegetable soup 202
tuna: cannellini beans and tuna salad 78
  onions stuffed with tuna 64
turnips 152–3
  glazed turnips 153
Tuscan cavolo nero soup 56

V
vegetable soup 202
vinegar 9
  leeks in a vinaigrette sauce 145
  peppers in a vinegary sauce 125

walnuts: celery, Gorgonzola and walnut salad 158
watercress: spinach and watercress soup 172
wild mushroom and pearl barley soup 94
wine: carrots braised in Marsala 34
  cauliflower stewed in wine 42
  fennel cooked in wine 87
  red cabbage cooked in wine 50
  sautéed mushrooms 93

Z
zucchini *see* courgettes

207

Acknowledgements

First and foremost, I must thank the Pavilion team, without whom this book would never have seen the light of the day. So, thank you Polly Powell and Katie Cowan for giving your consent to the publication; thank you Stephanie Milner, for giving me the right guidance and suggestions; and thank you Fiona Holman and Caitlin Leydon for checking and correcting my original manuscript. The designer, Laura Russell, and the photographer, Laura Edwards, with the help of the stylists, Tabitha Hawkins, Valerie Berry and Alex Gray, have managed to make the book look so beautiful and stylish. So many thanks to you all. A special thanks to Komal Patel, my dedicated publicity girl, for her invaluable contribution. And my most grateful thanks are for Vivien Green, my devoted literary agent, always there at the other end of the telephone for advice, suggestions, encouragement.

Now I must also thank my family next door, Julia and Charles and their children, Nellie, Johnny, Coco and Kate, for tasting many of my dishes and putting up with my endless asking, 'Was it good? Does it need more nutmeg? What would you like to change?' and all that. And thank you, Julia, for testing some of the recipes.

My deep thanks are also for some other members of my family and for some friends: for my son Guy and his Italian wife Giovanna and for my son Paul, always ready to calm me down and spur me on, and for my brother Marco for his culinary suggestions; for Myriam de'Castiglioni, Michelle Berriedale-Johnson, Freda Litton, Vicky Straker, Roger and Val Jupe, Bill and Margaretta Dacombe, Genista and Michael Toland, Gay Wilson, David and Simone Seckers, the owners and the staff of Abbotts, my local greengrocer in Shaftesbury. In one way or another, all of you have contributed to the writing of this book. Thank you.

I hope I remembered to thank everybody. If I forgot somebody, the somebody will have to forgive me and blame my old age.

Publisher's acknowledgements

Photography by Laura Edwards
Illustration by Alison Legg